Caribbean Diseases

Doctor George Low's expedition in 1901–02

Gordon C Cook

MD, DSc, FRCP, FRCPE, FRACP, FLS

Visiting Professor
University College London

Radcliffe Publishing
Oxford • New York

Radcliffe Publishing Ltd
18 Marcham Road
Abingdon
Oxon OX14 1AA
United Kingdom

www.radcliffe–oxford.com
Electronic catalogue and worldwide online ordering facility.

British Library Cataloguing in Publication Data

A catalogue record for this book is available from the British Library.

ISBN-13: 978 184619 345 3

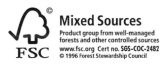

The paper used for the text pages of this book is FSC certified. FSC (The Forest Stewardship Council) is an international network to promote responsible management of the world's forests.

Mixed Sources
Product group from well-managed forests and other controlled sources
www.fsc.org Cert no. SGS-COC-2482
© 1996 Forest Stewardship Council

Typeset by Phoenix Photosetting, Chatham, Kent
Printed and bound by TJI Digital, Padstow, Cornwall, UK

Contents

Preface

The overriding *raison d'etre* of this book is to document (in George Carmichael Low's words) a 1901–02 expedition to the Caribbean (centred on the Windward Islands) which recorded accurately, probably for the first time, the disease spectrum (including parasites and their vectors) in that geographical location. Low was therefore a major pioneer (albeit a grossly underrated one) of a rapidly expanding specialty and his correspondence with Dr (later Sir) Patrick Manson (1844–1922) – then Medical Advisor to the Colonial Office – (transcribed here for the first time) does much to confirm his influence on the evolution of the specialty. The letters illustrate Manson's direction of Low's researches, and thus many of the thought processes of 'the father of tropical medicine' himself.[1] The correspondence also emphasises the importance of a knowledge of epidemiology and ecology to the early clinical parasitologists.

There were, of course, older records of disease in the West Indies, but most lack precision. Thus, Hans Sloane (1660–1753) had documented some of the diseases of Jamaica in his book: *Of the diseases I observed in Jamaica, and the Methods by which I used to Cure them*; he described yaws, elephantiasis and sleeping sickness in African slaves. Others of the early pioneers of 'medicine in the tropics' had also given accounts of diseases encountered in circumscribed localities. Thus, William Hillary (17??–63) and James Grainger (1721–66) had described the disease spectrum in Barbados and St Kitts, respectively.[2]

Low sent 31 letters to Manson (12 January 1901–02 April 1902), which were extant in 1993. They contain accounts of observations made during this period; many were epidemiological, but he also devoted a great deal of time sectioning mosquitoes in an attempt to delineate complete life-cycles; *Filaria demarquayi* (now designated *Mansonella ozzardi*) and *Filaria ozzardi*[3] were of particular interest. Manson (founder of the London School of Tropical Medicine [LSTM] and originator of the specialty), considered that both *F demarquayi* and *F perstans* were important helminths in a human context. [Looked at in retrospect it was, of course, unfortunate that Low spent so much time working on two filaria species which, it has transpired, have little clinical importance for *Homo sapiens*;

however, he was also able to accumulate a vast amount of other scientific data.] He also confirmed the causative association between *Filaria bancrofti* and elephantiasis, which was known to Manson at Amoy, China in 1877.[4] A later project was to assist in the elimination of malaria and yellow fever by draining swamps and other areas containing stagnant water. He mentioned in the correspondence to Manson that he had communicated with (Sir) Ronald Ross (1857–1932), (whose major research on malaria transmission had been undertaken a mere 4–5 years before) on the best methods and practicability of eradicating malaria from various Caribbean islands.

Low also recorded the presence or absence of various diseases on various West Indian islands; for example, he documented cases of typhoid, yaws, smallpox, yellow fever and many other infective entities which before the antimicrobial era were untreatable.

All of these letters from Low to Manson from British possessions in the Caribbean were until recently in the Manuscript Collection of the London School of Hygiene and Tropical Medicine, although they are presently 'missing'. Chapters 4–9 are transcripts of the original letters with the exception that I have italicised the names of helminths and insects, and have highlighted the major diseases in bold font. My editing throughout has however been minimal. These documents also provide a great deal to knowledge of disease causation and prevention in the early days of the LSTM – which had been founded in 1899 – and also the formal discipline *tropical medicine*.

Low's primary ambition was thus to elucidate the complete life-cycles of previously poorly documented filarial infection(s).[5] However, his expedition became increasingly oriented towards *prevention* (in the wake of Manson's, Ross' and Walter Reed's recent pioneering discoveries).[6] Thus the correspondence contains much on *prevention* of both malaria and yellow fever, and also attempts to convince the lay public resident in the Caribbean, that mosquitoes must be eliminated from the environment. Another objective was to collect both helminths and entomological specimens for the LSTM. Low therefore helped enormously to place the new discipline on a *scientific* basis.

Mary Gibson kindly drew my attention to the Low–Manson correspondence (previously unpublished) which was in the Manuscript Collection of the Library of the London School of Hygiene and Tropical Medicine. I am grateful also to Mr Robert N Smark (Keeper of Muniments at the University of St Andrews) and Dr G O Cowan OBE for making available extant information on Low's undergraduate career. Jo Currie, Assistant Librarian of the Special Collections at Edinburgh University Library, provided material on Low's years at that University. Amberley Moore, Honorary Secretary of the British Ornithologists' Club, kindly supplied information regarding Low's involvement with ornithology.

G C Cook

April 2009

References and Notes

1 P Manson-Bahr. *History of the School of Tropical Medicine in London (1899–1949).* London: H K Lewis 1956: 328; G C Cook. *From the Greenwich Hulks to Old St Pancras: a history of tropical disease in London.* London: Athlone Press 1992: 338. [*See also:* P Manson-Bahr. *The Manson Saga. Trans R Soc trop Med Hyg* 1945; 38: 401–17. G C Cook. *Disease in the Merchant Navy: a history of the Seamen's Hospital Society.* Oxford: Radcliffe Publishing 2007: 630; J W W Stephens, M P Sutphen. Manson, Sir Patrick (1844–1922). In: H C G Matthew, B Harrison (eds). *Oxford Dictionary of National Biography.* Oxford: Oxford University Press: 2004; 36: 553–5.]

2 *Op cit.* See Note 1 above (Cook, 1992). [*See also:* G C Cook. *Tropical Medicine: an illustrated history of the pioneers.* London: Academic Press 2007: 14–16.]

3 **Albert Tronson Ozzard** (??–1929) qualified (MRCS, LSA) from the London Hospital Medical College in 1887. He subsequently served at Suddie, British Guiana (now Guyana) from 1887 until 1927. His research publications were on malaria, filariasis, and ankylostomiasis. [*See also*: *Medical Directory.* London: J & A Churchill 1908; 1582.]

4 *Op cit.* See Note 2 above (Cook, 2007) 53–5.

5 J J C Buckley. On the development, in *Culicoides furens* Poey, of *Filaria* (= *Mansonella*) *ozzardi* Manson 1897. *J Helminthol* 1934; 12: 99–118; D I Grove. *A History of Human Helminthology.* Wallingford, UK: CAB International 1990: 734–6.

6 *Op cit.* See Note 2 above (Cook 2007; 53–5, 88–92, 105–8). [*See also*: G Williams. *The Plague Killers.* New York: Charles Scribner's Sons 1969: 345.]

Prologue

'Tropical medicine' as a distinct discipline came into being during a 20–year period (1894–1914) and is sometimes equated with 'colonial medicine'. Low himself has outlined the origin(s) of the discipline, which arguably began with Manson's demonstration of the man-mosquito component in the life-cycle of *Filaria nocturna* (*Wuchereria bancrofti*) in 1877.[1]

Thus the formal discipline was in 1901, when Low set out on this expedition, in its infancy. Ross' discoveries in India, which demonstrated scientifically that mosquitoes were involved in malaria (*Plasmodium* and *Proteosoma*) transmission had been carried out as recently as 1897 and 1898. These exciting events were therefore fresh in the minds – not only of the pioneers of the discipline – but in those of the lay public generally.[2] Implication of another species of mosquito – *Aëdes aegypti* – in the transmission of yellow fever by the American Yellow Fever Commission was not accomplished until late 1900, and the results were not widely known until February 1901 – i.e. *during* Low's expedition.[3]

However, the aetiology of most tropical diseases was in 1901–02 still undetermined. It was not until 1903, for example, that the causative agent of the 'negro lethargy' was identified. At about the same time, the cause of Kala-azar (visceral leishmaniasis) was also determined.[4]

This was thus an extremely exciting time; clinical parasitology was fast developing, and Low (working at Manson's school – the London School of Tropical Medicine) was at the forefront of activity.[5]

References and Notes

1   G C Cook. *Tropical Medicine: an illustrated history of the pioneers*. London: Academic Press 2007: 53–5.
2   *Ibid*. 81–102. [*See also*: G C Cook. Mosquito involvement in the malaria life cycle. *J Med Biog* 1998; 6: 182–3.]

3 *Ibid*. 103–13. [*See also*: H H Scott. *A History of Tropical Medicine*. London: Edward Arnold 1939: 279–453; G Williams. *The Plague Killers*. New York: Charles Scribner's Sons 1969: 345.]

4 *Ibid*. 153–4, 177–82.

5 F E G Cox (ed). *The Wellcome Trust Illustrated History of Tropical Diseases*. London: The Wellcome Trust 1996: 452. [*See also*: G C Cook. *From the Greenwich Hulks to Old St Pancras: a history of tropical disease in London*. London: Athlone Press 1992: 338; G C Cook. *Disease in the Merchant Navy: a history of the Seamen's Hospital Society*. Oxford: Radcliffe Publishing 2007: 630.]

Chapter 1

George Carmichael Low (1872–1952)

Who was George Low? George Carmichael Low (Figure 1.1), the third son of Samuel Miller Low (master manufacturer of flax machinery), was born at Monifieth, South Forfarshire, on 14 October, 1872. Little is known of his early life. Having graduated in arts (MA on 14 April 1892) at Madras College, St Andrews (extant records are incomplete), he went on to a highly successful undergraduate and early postgraduate medical career at Edinburgh University. Figure 1.2 shows two pages from his entry in the medical student schedule, and Figure 1.3 shows the Edinburgh Medical School in 1896. He subsequently held house appointments at the Edinburgh Royal Infirmary;[1] Figure 1.4 shows the residents (including Low) in 1898. His MD thesis (229 pages) was entitled 'Human filariasis'; he was awarded the University's Gold Medal in Tropical Medicine in 1912.

In November 1899, Low joined Dr (later Sir) Patrick Manson immediately after the London School of Tropical Medicine (LSTM) had been founded at the Albert Dock Hospital (ADH) London.[2] Shortly afterwards, he travelled to Heidelberg and Vienna to learn a technique for sectioning mosquitoes in celloidin using a sliding microtome. Immediately after return to London, he used this technique to examine alcohol-preserved *Culex fatigans* which had fed on individuals infected with *Filaria* (now *Wuchereria) bancrofti* in Brisbane, Queensland, which had been sent to Manson by Thomas Bancroft (1860–1933). Demonstration (on 24 March 1900) of filariae in the entire length of the proboscis sheath led to an obvious conclusion that man is infected by larval filariae via a mosquito bite.[3] (At that time human infection was widely believed to occur via mosquito-contaminated water, and Manson himself subscribed to this view.)

In the autumn of 1900, Low, together with L W Sambon, an artist, and a servant, spent three months on the Roman Campagna in a region highly endemic for *Plasmodium vivax* infection. One hour before sunset

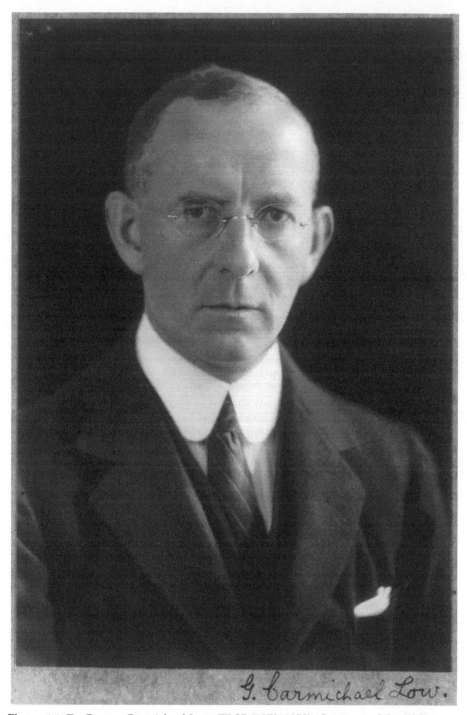

Figure 1.1: Dr George Carmichael Low, FRCP (1872–1952). Courtesy of the Wellcome Library, London (reproduced with permission).

each day they 'imprisoned' themselves in a mosquito-proof hut, where they remained until dawn, thereby escaping mosquito bites and, as a result, clinical malaria. During that expedition, *P vivax*-infected mosquitoes were dispatched to London, where they were allowed to infect P T Manson (son of Patrick), a medical student at Guy's Hospital, and also Warren, a laboratory technician. Both developed clinical malaria, which was eventually cured with quinine.[4] These two pieces of clinical investigation established beyond doubt that *human* malaria is contracted by the bite of mosquitoes (the controversy concerning priority in this discovery will not be spelled out here, but has recently been reviewed).[5]

This book documents Low's contributions during the period January 1901 to April 1902. In 1901, he travelled to the West Indies (the Windward Islands and British Guiana), where he both confirmed Manson's work linking *Filaria bancrofti* with elephantiasis, and made numerous observations on other human filarial infections. He also became increasingly interested in *prevention* of both malaria and yellow fever.

Shortly after his return to London in May 1902, Low headed the Royal Society's first sleeping-sickness expedition (accompanied by A Castellani and C Christie) to Entebbe, Uganda – on the northern shore of Lake Victoria Nyanza – in order to investigate the cause of a large and severe epidemic of the 'negro lethargy'. This expedition could have been a triumphant success, because Castellani actually demonstrated *Trypanosoma* sp in patients with the disease (sleeping sickness); however he became obsessed with an idea developed by Portuguese workers, that *Streptococcus* sp was responsible. It fell to D Bruce (and D N Nabarro) to clinch the *Trypanosoma* sp theory shortly afterwards.[6]

Returning again to London in 1903, Low had already become a towering figure in tropical medicine; when the post of superintendent of the ADH became vacant, he was the obvious choice.[7] He was apparently an excellent teacher and organiser, and remained at the School and Hospital for virtually the whole of his subsequent professional life. In 1918 he was appointed physician, and in 1919 senor physician, to the ADH.[8] During the Great War (1914–18) he became a major in the Indian Medical Service, treating officers with tropical diseases at the ADH. In 1920, the LSTM moved to Endsleigh Gardens, London WC1, and Low became senior physician of the Hospital for Tropical Diseases (HTD) which until 1929 was housed in the same building as the School. When the London School of Hygiene and Tropical Medicine (LSHTM) was founded in 1924, Low became Director of the Division of Clinical Tropical

UNIVERSITY OF EDINBURGH.

DEGREES IN MEDICINE.

PRELIMINARY EXAMINATION AND COURSE OF STUDY.

N.B.—*Before filling in the Entries required, please to read over the Directions on page 4.*

Candidate's Name in full, *George Carmichael Low M.A*

Birthplace and Date of Birth.	Of what Country.	ADDRESSES AT THE DATES OF ENTERING FOR THE FIRST, SECOND, AND FINAL PROFESSIONAL EXAMINATIONS.	
		Edinburgh Address.	Home Address.
Monifieth 14th Oct. 1872.	*Scotland.*	*8 Eyre Crescent*	*Ashlea Monifieth*

PRELIMINARY EXAMINATION.

Board or Boards at which Preliminary Examination passed, or University by which Degree in Arts conferred, as the case may be.	Date or Dates of Examination, or of Degree in Arts.	Preliminary Subjects Passed.	Date of Registration as a Student of Medicine.
St Andrews University	*15th april 1892*	✓ *M.A.*	*May 2nd 1892.*
			✓

COURSE OF STUDY.

See Directions, page 4.

Class.	No. of Lectures in the Course.	Date of the Course.	Teacher's Name.	Name of University.	Name of Medical School.	Fee paid to Extra-Academical Teacher in Edinburgh or in Glasgow.
Subjects of First Professional Examination.						
Botany	✓ 50	*May 2nd 1892.*	*Prof. Balfour*	*Edinburgh*		
Natural History	✓ 50	*May 7th 1892*	*Prof. Ewart*	*Edinburgh*		
Chemistry	✓ 100	*1892-93*	*Prof. C Brown*	*Edinburgh*		
Practical Chemistry	✓ 50	*1892-93*	" " "	"		

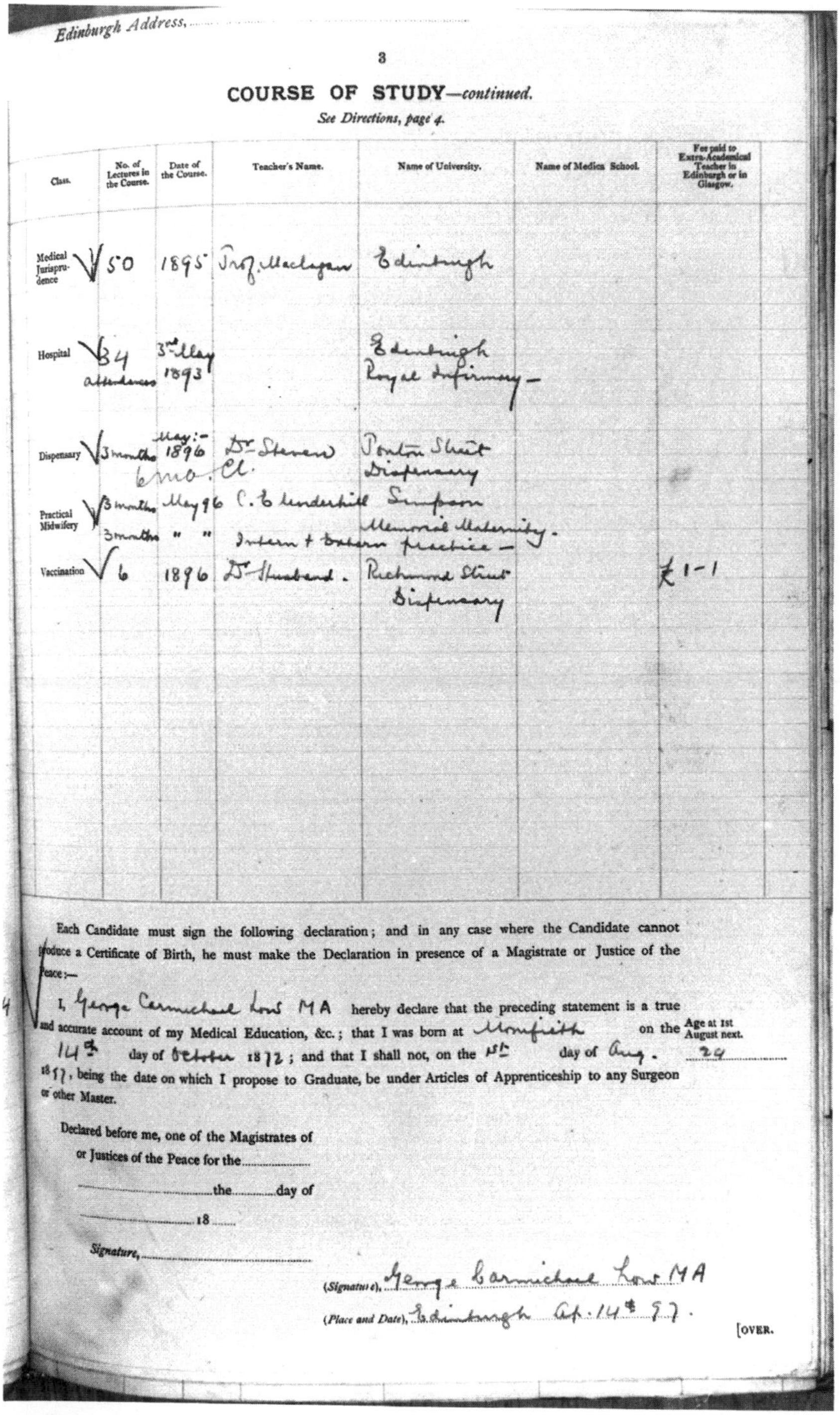

Edinburgh Address,

3

COURSE OF STUDY—*continued.*

See Directions, page 4.

Class.	No. of Lectures in the Course.	Date of the Course.	Teacher's Name.	Name of University.	Name of Medical School.	Fee paid to Extra-Academical Teacher in Edinburgh or in Glasgow.
Medical Jurisprudence	√ 50	1895	Prof. Maclagan	Edinburgh		
Hospital	√ 84 attendances	3rd May 1893		Edinburgh Royal Infirmary —		
Dispensary	√ 3 months 6 mo. Cl.	May:- 1896	Dr. Stevens	Ponton Street Dispensary		
Practical Midwifery	√ 3 months 3 months	May 96 "	C. E. Underhill "	Simpson Memorial Maternity. Intern + Extern practice —		
Vaccination	√ 6	1896	Dr. Husband.	Richmond Street Dispensary		£1-1

Each Candidate must sign the following declaration; and in any case where the Candidate cannot produce a Certificate of Birth, he must make the Declaration in presence of a Magistrate or Justice of the Peace:—

I, George Carmichael Low MA hereby declare that the preceding statement is a true and accurate account of my Medical Education, &c.; that I was born at Monifieth on the 14th day of October 1872; and that I shall not, on the 1st day of Aug. 1897, being the date on which I propose to Graduate, be under Articles of Apprenticeship to any Surgeon or other Master. Age at 1st August next. 24

Declared before me, one of the Magistrates of or Justices of the Peace for the............

..................the..........day of

..................18......

Signature,..................

(*Signature*), George Carmichael Low MA

(*Place and Date*), Edinburgh Ap. 14th 97.

[OVER.

Figure 1.2 a, b: Pages 1 and 3 of Low's entry in the Edinburgh University medical student schedule – referring to some subjects in the Final Professional Examination. Page 3 contains a declaration signed by Low on 14 April 1897.

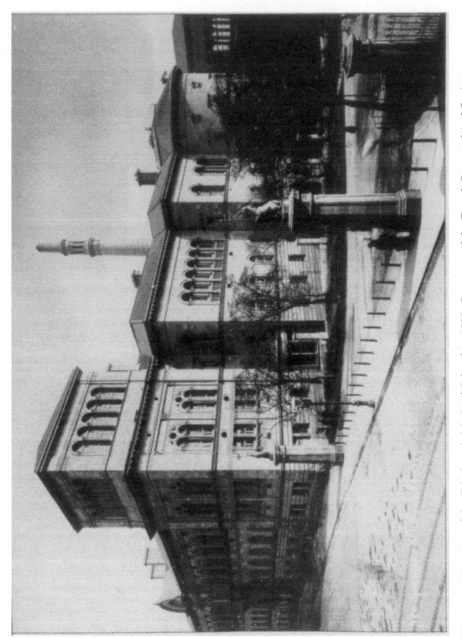

Figure 1.3: Exterior of the Edinburgh Medical School in 1880. Courtesy of the Royal Geographical Society (reproduced with permission).

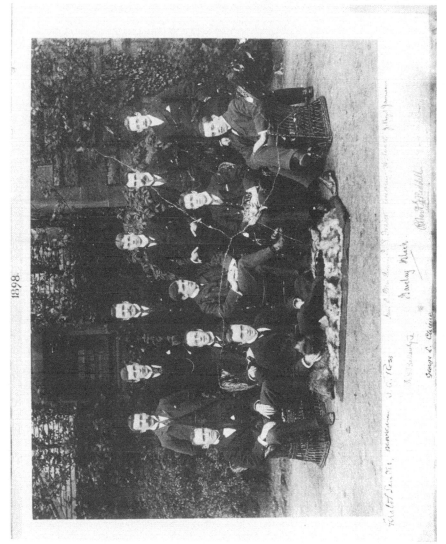

Figure 1.4: Residents of the Royal Infirmary, Edinburgh, in 1898; Low is at the extreme right of the front row.

Medicine.[9] He later carried out a great deal of clinical research in London into many tropical diseases, including tropical sprue[10] (Figure 1.5).

In 1907 he was the joint founder (with Mr [later Sir] James Cantlie [1851–1926]) of the (Royal) Society of Tropical Medicine and Hygiene, and during his presidency in 1931 was responsible for the removal of this itinerant society to Manson House, Portland Place, London W1 – where it remained until 2003. In 1994, HRH the Princess Royal officially opened the George Carmichael Low auditorium (at Manson House), which had recently been refurbished.[11]

Elected FRCP in 1924, Low also received Edinburgh University's Straits Settlements Gold Medal, the Mary Kingsley Medal of the Liverpool School of Tropical Medicine, and was also appointed a *Membre d'Honneur* of the *Société Belge de Medicine Tropicale,* and a corresponding member of the *Société de Pathologie Exotique,* Paris.

He was also one of the most notable ornithologists of his day (*see* below), and wrote extensively on this subject. He was, in fact, one of a group of bird-watchers who put London's ornithology on the map; he held high office in the British Ornithologists' Club (BOC) (*see* below

[Q. J. M., July, 1928.]

523

SPRUE

AN ANALYTICAL STUDY OF 150 CASES[1]

By G. CARMICHAEL LOW

(From the Hospital for Tropical Diseases, London)

I KNOW of no better definition for sprue than that given by Sir Patrick Manson, in his *Tropical Diseases,* sixth edition, 1917, page 549 : ' By the term " sprue " is understood a peculiar and very dangerous form of chronic catarrhal inflammation of the whole or part of the alimentary canal, generally associated with disturbance of the chologenic function of the liver and, probably, of the functions of the other glandular organs subserving digestion. Although a disease of warm climates, it may develop for the first time in temperate climates ; only, however, in individuals who have previously resided in the tropics or sub-tropics.'

Figure 1.5: Beginning of an article analysing 150 cases of tropical sprue (G C Low. *Quart J Med* 1928; 21: 523–34).

and Figure 1.6), was a Member of Council of the Zoological Society and Royal Society for the Protection of Birds (RSPB), and became official bird-watcher at Kensington Gardens (*see* below) – where he must have often passed the Speke Memorial, commemorating the discovery of the source of the Nile at Lake Victoria Nyanza, where his sleeping-sickness expedition had taken him.[12]

Low thus made enormous contributions to British tropical medicine during its 'golden era'. Why did he receive so little official recognition? Unlike many of his contemporaries who achieved far greater fame, he devoted most of his life to the LSTM and the HTD; time spent abroad was therefore limited. He made major research contributions, however, and his teaching and administrative achievements were of inestimable value. In many ways he was the natural successor to Sir Patrick Manson (1844–1922), and as a result lived in the shadow of the 'father of tropical medicine'. He died on 31 July 1952 in London.[13] He had married Edith Nash in 1906, but there were no children of the marriage. Sir Philip Manson-Bahr (1881–1966) later compared Low with Manson:

> [he] had many links with Patrick Manson not only as a brother Scot, but also through friendly family associations. He was brought up in a strictly disciplined atmosphere, absorbing much local lore from sporting and naturalistic sources during his youth and these trends and traits, so redolent of his family, remained dominant features throughout his long life.[14]

Manson-Bahr also wrote of Low's days at the LSTM and the HTD, where he spent most of his career:

> On returning to London he was the obvious choice for the post of third Superintendent of the [LSTM] in succession to Dr. C W Daniels [*see* Chapter 4] who had resigned. He was admirably adapted to this position as he had a considerable flair for organization and had the reputation of a good disciplinarian. He possessed a large store of accurate and well documented information and made an admirable teacher. He had a rather *stuccato*, stilted style and was apt at times to be pawky and doctrinaire, but the class soon learned that he meant what he said. He was punctilious and assiduous in his duties and the school progressed under his tutelage. He was succeeded in 1905 by Daniels on his return from Malaya. For a short period he left the

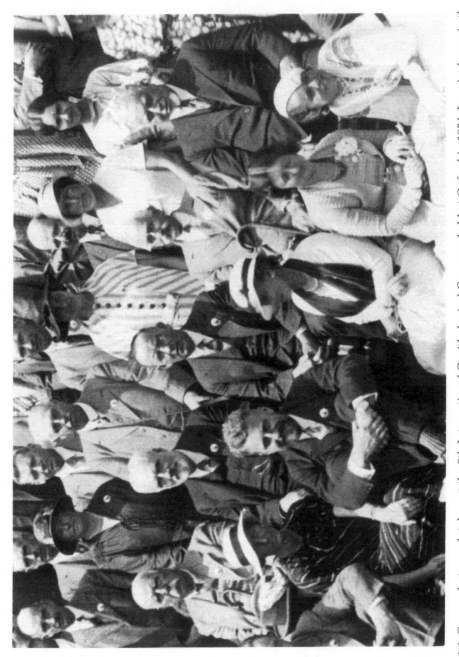

Figure 1.6: Group photograph taken at the 8th International Ornithological Congress held at Oxford in 1934; Low is shown in the centre of the second row. Courtesy of the Natural History Museum, London (reproduced with permission).

school to become pathologist to the West London Hospital, but in 1910 he was appointed physician to the [ADH] and assisted Manson [with] his clinical demonstrations. Henceforward his work was centred in the Metropolis. As senior physician to the [HTD], and as Director of the Clinical Division [at the LSHTM], he followed the school to Endsleigh Gardens in 1920 and to the new [LSHTM] in 1929, retiring on the age limit in 1937.

Manson-Bahr continued with his reminiscences of Low as a physician:

Low had many endearing personal peculiarities. He clung firmly to his Scottish traditions. Erect, robust, of medium height with coal-black hair which never became bleached, and bearing himself with rather an assertive carriage and with a florid countenance, he would greet his friends with a recurrent wag of the head and a cheery 'How's yoursell?'. To a reciprocal reply he would utter 'Eh Eh Eh, Good, good'. He often affected a clipped, halting style, giving the impression that his attention had been diverted elsewhere, but the twinkle of one eye with a particularly attractive smile would reassure listeners that he had returned to earth. His clinics were always the subject of much attention and no little amusement. Many would crowd into the theatre to enjoy the fun. Who can forget the recital of the forty-seven causes of enlargements of the spleen and his insistence on taking a particularly meticulous history of the case with reference to previous illnesses and the great astonishment when another was added to this list; the last being an ovarian cyst which was mistaken for a spleen. Sometimes a facetious fraction of the class would try to trap him; once, it will be remembered, by the substitution of one patient with a glass eye and another with a wooden leg in which he was induced to test their reflexes. On occasions he could be quite argumentative and combative. It is related that on his first attempt at the M.R.C.P. examination an argument arose upon the Scots pronunciation of Kakke, a native name for beri-beri, which the examiners could neither understand nor appreciate. He took this as a slight upon his country and thus unfortunately he was deferred.

He also recalled that Low was something of a wit, albeit sometimes subconsciously:

He was possessed of many Scottish witticisms which emerged at odd and unexpected moments. He himself had a quite unconscious humour which made the scene even more hilarious. When at a loss for a word he would substitute 'the thing' and expressions such as 'where is the thing' (which might be a patient or pathological specimen) or 'Have you seen the thing' (which might be a parasite or an appendix) would occasionally escape him.

Few who were present can ever forget the occasion when he was asked to unveil a commemorative tablet in the hall of the [HTD]. In order to give point to the story it should be stated that a test court case of the legal meaning of the patent name 'Tabloid' was then being waged by Messrs. Burroughs, Wellcome, and that the Wellcome Research Institution was our nextdoor neighbour.[15] 'Ladies and gentlemen,' he unconcernedly exclaimed, 'I will now proceed to unveil the 'tabloid'.' No one was more astonished than himself at the outburst of laughter from the audience.

From his long association with the school and his influence on its infancy and adolescence Low impressed his personality on the students and as such he will long be remembered.

However, Manson-Bahr has also pointed out that Low's judgement was not *always* correct:

Once the author had under his care a patient from Assam lying very ill with kala azar and, as is usual as the disease progressed, so she became progressively more pigmented, especially on the hands and feet. He expressed a desire to examine the case and so he was conducted into the room by the Sister in charge. His first remark was 'How long is it since her face were washed?' The Sister flared up, saying – 'You should know, Dr Low, that this is done here every morning.' 'I don't believe it,' he vigorously answered, 'bring me a basin of water, soap and a scrubbing brush. I once recollect,' he said, 'seeing Manson convert a *Tinea nigra* into a *Tinea alba* in this manner.' But this time the spell did not work for the blackness still remained, so he was nonplussed, but blurted out, 'I suppose you really were born like that.'[16]

The Times considered:

> Low was one of the young 'doctor naturalists' who were brought forward by Manson.[17]

Sir Neil Hamilton Fairley FRS wrote of him as:

> An accurate observer and methodical to an unusual degree. … A sound physician and clinical teacher [who] possessed a profound knowledge of Tropical Medicine in its geographical, biological and pathological aspects. … A man of great intellectual honesty, said what he thought and adopted a justifiably critical and somewhat conservative attitude to things medical which were 'not proved'.[18]

An anonymous obituary probably also written by Manson-Bahr (*see* above) in the *British Medical Journal* claimed that after his appointment as Superintendent of the LSTM:

> He found himself chained to the Metropolis, spending the rest of his career in the service of the School and as Physician to the [HTD].[19]

Low the Ornithologist

Low was to become Vice-Chairman of the BOC (1938–39), having served as Honorary Secretary/Treasurer from 1923–29 and Honorary Secretary from 1943–45. He edited the Club's *Bulletin* from 1930–35 and 1940–45, as well as being a regular contributor.[20]

In a notice in *Ibis* (the Bulletin of the British Ornithologists' Club) in 1953, Manson-Bahr (himself a distinguished ornithologist) recalled:

> There always existed, deeply hidden, a latent love of natural history in his make-up. He possessed a tidy mind and was able to correlate and store up knowledge in an amazing manner. At one time he took up the study of trees and mesmerized his guests by reeling off the botanical names of most of those in Kew, but about 1920 [when around 50] his leanings to ornithology became dominant and he joined the B.O.C. and became a constant companion of the most prominent ornithologists of that day – Hartert, Percy Lowe, Norman Kinnear, Bannerman, Witherby, Mathews, Meinertzhagen and many others. Soon,

too, there appeared his first serious contribution to scientific ornithology in the 'Literature of the Charadriiformes' (1924), of which a second edition appeared in 1931. At the same time he undertook the section on 'Aves' for the centenary volume of the Zoological Society [of London] in 1929. Only one with the most methodical mind could have completed such meticulous compilations at one and the same time. ...

No account of Low's life would be complete without some reference to his work as a bird-watcher [*see* above]. He was one of the band which frequented Staines and other reservoirs at week-ends. On these occasions he was a familiar figure with his telescope, and will long be remembered for his scotticisms and enthusiasms, as when he spotted Bewick's Swans and Red-throated Divers on the Serpentine or Golden-eye on the Round Pond in Kensington Gardens. With Holte-Macpherson he made solid contributions to the ornithology of London and will be missed as much in his haunts as in the Bird Room at South Kensington.

At one time Low was a keen shot and ran a 'market-garden' partridge shoot somewhere along the Great West Road. There, after many attempts, he bagged a White-fronted Goose one February evening, and the writer well remembers the remarks of his gun-bearer on that occasion: 'I'd sooner be in the condemned cell in Reading Gaol, Sir, than 'ave 'im after me with that gun of 'is'. For many years he was on the Council of the Zoological Society and the R.S.P.B. ... [21]

Barclay-Smith also recorded the following reminiscences of Low as an ornithologist:

At the close of the 9th International Ornithological Congress in Rouen in 1938 the majority of participants joined an expedition to the Camargue. Some remained longer, and these included the Scottish trio [Low, W G Glegg – a brewer, and A Holte-Macpherson – a director of Watneys Brewery] and myself. It was an unforgettable experience; on excursions they each carried a telescope and umbrella and there were often arguments as to where a picnic lunch should be. Carmichael Low once finally authoritatively ordered us on to what turned out to be an ant-heap.

And, going back two years:

> It was announced on the Agenda of the meeting of the [BOC] on 12 February 1936 that Dr. Carmichael Low would give a short description of his recent tour round the world with the British Medical Association and an account of some of the more interesting birds seen on the journey. He told us that 'the trip was a wonderful one in every way and lasted from July 1934 to November 1935, over 240 species and sub-species being recorded'. He showed a large number of pictures on the epidiascope and though the majority of these showed lovely girls sitting under sun-umbrellas, he was quite oblivious to the amusement he thus evoked. At the meeting on 24 October 1942 he exhibited an Andean Gull, which he explained had 'survived for a little over 4 years in the London Zoo and died eventually of congestion and oedema of the lungs', adding that he had 'got' the body which he proceeded to pass round on a plate.

And finally, an anecdote which has for long apparently been remembered by members of the BOC:

> Story has it that during the last war [1939–45] Low was leaving the Natural History Museum when an air-raid warning sounded, at which he promptly opened his umbrella.[22]

Conclusion(s)

Low therefore contributed enormously to the formal discipline of Tropical Medicine – which was rapidly emerging at the turn of the century.[23] He was an outstanding teacher and administrator who was in many respects the lynch-pin of the *clinical* discipline in London. Some of his early research was clearly of the highest calibre. His greatest overall contribution was arguably, however, to the (Royal) Society of Tropical Medicine and Hygiene; in addition to enormous service to the Society, including its removal to Manson House, he rescued it financially in its early days, and donated both the rostrum – which remained in place until 2003 – and the gavel, in December and June 1931 respectively. However, Low did not receive a civil award and there are many now, including some within the discipline of Tropical

Medicine, who are not even familiar with his name, let alone his numerous achievements.

Why was Low underrated both then and now? He certainly served in the 'shadow' of Manson, and this may not have assisted him! Unlike the majority of pioneers in this discipline, he spent only a short time (some two to three years) serving in a tropical environment, whereas most major figures had devoted the bulk of their careers to practice and research in a 'warm climate'. But these facts are inadequate to explain why so little is generally known about George Carmichael Low.

References and Notes

1 Anonymous. Obituary: Dr G Carmichael Low. *Times, Lond.* 1 August 1952: 8; Anonymous. Obituary: George Carmichael Low. *Lancet* 1952; ii: 296–7; Anonymous. Obituary: George Carmichael Low. *Br med J* 1952; ii: 341–2; N H Fairley. George Carmichael Low. *Trans R Soc trop Med Hyg* 1952; 46: 571–3; P Manson-Bahr. Dr George Carmichael Low, MA, MD, CM, FRCP. 1872–1952. In: *History of the School of Tropical Medicine in London (1899–1949).* London: H K Lewis 1956: 158–62; Anonymous. Low, George Carmichael. *Who Was Who 1951–1960.* London: A & C Black 1961: 677; G C Cook. George Carmichael Low FRCP: twelfth President of the Society and underrated pioneer of tropical medicine. *Trans R Soc trop Med Hyg* 1993; 87: 355–60; G C Cook. George Carmichael Low FRCP: an underrated figure in British tropical medicine. *J R Coll Phys Lond* 1993; 27: 81–2; M Worboys. Low, George Carmichael (1872–1952). In: H C G Matthew, B Harrison (eds). *Oxford Dictionary of National Biography.* Oxford: Oxford University Press 2004; 34: 550–1; G C Cook. *Tropical Medicine: an illustrated history of the pioneers.* London: Academic Press 2007: 127–143; Anonymous. Low, George Carmichael. *Munks Roll;* 4: 594–5.

2 G C Cook. *From the Greenwich Hulks to Old St Pancras: a history of tropical disease in London.* London: Athlone Press 1992: 337. [*See also*: G C Cook, A J Webb. The Albert Dock Hospital, London: the original site (in 1899) of Tropical Medicine as a new discipline. *Acta Trop* 2001; 79: 249–55; *Op cit.* See Note 1 above (Cook 2007; 57–60).]

3 G C Low. A recent observation on *Filaria nocturna* in *Culex*: probable mode of infection of man. *Br med J* 1900; i: 1456–7.

4 P Manson. Experimental proof of the mosquito-malaria theory. *Br med J* 1900; ii: 949–51. [*See also*: L J Bruce-Chwatt. Three hundred and fifty years of the Peruvian bark. *Br med J* 1988; i: 1486–7.]

5 *Op cit.* See Note 1 above (Cook 2007).

6 G C Cook. Correspondence from Dr George Carmichael Low to Dr Patrick Manson during the first Ugandan sleeping sickness expedition. *J med Biog* 1993; 1: 215–29.

7 *Op cit.* See Notes 1 (Fairley) and 2 above.

8 G C Cook. *Disease in the Merchant Navy: a history of the Seamen's Hospital Society*. Oxford: Radcliffe Publishing 2007: 630. [*See also:* Note 2 above.]

9 *Op cit.* See Note 2 above.

10 G C Low. Sprue: an analytical study of 150 cases. *Quart J Med* 1928; 21: 523–34.

11 *Op cit.* See Note 1 above (Cook, 2007).

12 *Ibid.*

13 *Op cit.* See Note 1 above.

14 *Op cit.* See Note 1 above (Manson-Bahr).

15 R R James. *Henry Wellcome.* London: Hodder and Stoughton 1994: 422.

16 *Op cit.* See Note 14 above.

17 *Op cit.* See Note 1 above (*Times*).

18 *Op cit.* See Note 1 above (Fairley).

19 *Op cit.* See Note 1 above (Anonymous *Br med J*).

20 P H Manson-Bahr. A short history of the Club. *Bulletin of the British Ornithologists' Club.* 71: 2–4.

21 P Manson-Bahr. Obituary: George Carmichael Low, M.A., M.D., C.M., F.R.C.P. *Ibis* 1953; 95: 140–2.

22 P Barclay-Smith. Recollections of personalities of the Club: G Carmichael Low. *Bulletin of the British Ornithologists' Club* 1980; 100: 19–20.

23 *Op cit.* See Note 1 above (Cook 1993, 2007).

Chapter 2

The Craggs prize, and the *Filaria demarquayi* dilemma

In May 1900, Low was awarded a scholarship by the London School of Tropical Medicine (LSTM), then administered by the Seamen's Hospital Society (SHS).[1] A memorandum published later by the SHS (in 1912) contained a short account of the prize, and of Low's appointment:

> THIS Prize owes its origin to the generosity of Sir John Craggs M.V.O.,[2] who, on the occasion of the Dinner presided over by Mr Joseph Chamberlain [1836–1914], in 1899 in connection with the foundation of the School, announced his intention to provide £300 per annum for a Travelling Scholarship for three years. At the expiration of that period he continued his benefaction by providing annually a prize of £50 for the Student of the London School of Tropical Medicine [LSTM] who in competition shows evidence of having made the most valuable contribution to the knowledge of Tropical Medicine during the year.
>
> The prize has been always eagerly competed for, and the work of deciding as to the merit of the papers sent in has often been a difficult one.
>
> It is not too much to say that the action of Sir John Craggs gave a stimulus to the School that has very largely conduced to the continuous success that has attended its labours.
>
> A perusal of the following memoranda in relation to the work of the successful Candidates and the knowledge that has accrued in the course of their investigations will convince, not only members of the profession, but the ordinary reader, of the vast benefit that has been conferred upon mankind by the establishment of this prize.
>
> The first investigator to be appointed in connection with Sir John Cragg's gift was Dr. G. C. Low, a Student of the School, who, at a meeting of Lecturers and Teachers in the School held in

May 1900, was unanimously elected Craggs Research Scholar, and forthwith arrangements were made for the research work which it was proposed to carry out during the three years of his Scholarship.

In the first instance it was decided to demonstrate without any possibility of doubt that malaria is carried from one patient to another by means of the mosquito [*see* Chapter 1], and accordingly it was decided to make an experiment in a malarious district. Dr. Louis Sambon, one of the Teachers in the Tropical School, and Mr. A. Engel Terzi, an artist, were associated with Dr. Low for this purpose, and the summer of 1900 they spent in the Roman Campagna.[3]

Filaria demarquayi

Manson himself wrote in 1897 that although he did not know what they were, he had no doubt that *F demarquayi* had undoubted pathological consequences. However, the following year C W Daniels (1862–1927) [*see* Chapter 4] considered that there was no evidence for a pathological role!

In 1891 Manson had described two new species of filaria – *Filaria diurna* (which causes loaiasis) and *Filaria perstans* (which he believed caused the 'negro lethargy' of East Africa); *F sanguinis hominis* or *F nocturna* (renamed *Wuchereria bancrofti*) had of course been known for many years, and this was the organism on which he had carried out his major research at Amoy, China. In 1897, on the basis of specimens sent to him in London by Newsham (*see* Chapter 4) of St Vincent, he concluded that there were a further *two* species:

> ... an entirely new filaria which at Blanchard's suggestion, I have named *filaria Demarquayi*. This new filaria is shaped exactly like *filaria nocturna* and *filaria diurna* but is very much smaller. I do not feel justified in giving the measurements of the dried organisms, the only specimens available, as in consequence of the shrivelling the parasites have undergone, the dimensions may be materially altered; suffice it to say that *filaria Demarquayi* is less than half the size of *filaria nocturna*. *Filaria Demarquayi* has no sheath, but, like *filaria perstans*, is naked in the blood ... it exhibits no diurnal periodicity

whatever, being present in the peripheral blood both during the day and during the night.

In the same year Manson had received some blood slides from Ozzard (*see* Preface) who was working in the 'interior' of British Guiana (now Guyana), and these contained two different microfilariae:

> One of these minute filariae closely resembled *filaria Demarquayi* of St Vincent, being minute and sharp-tailed and without a sheath; the other closely resembled, if ... not identical with, *filaria perstans* a parasite which hitherto I had found only in West African blood.

Manson concluded:

> *I do think* [author's italics] the sharp-tailed Demerara filaria [the one found in British Guiana] is a new species and not identical with *filaria Demarquayi* ... this new filaria of Demerara ... I propose to call provisionally *filaria Ozzardi*.[4]

However Daniels (*see* above) was less certain that this represented a *new* species, and Otho Galgey (*see* Chapter 4), colonial assistant surgeon in St Lucia, concluded that the two worms were identical:

> I am inclined to believe that all are *filaria Demarquayii* [sic]; that is to say, that the *filaria Demarquayii* [sic] of St. Vincent, and that discovered by me in St. Lucia, and the sharp-tailed form of *filaria Ozzardi* (British Guiana) are identical.[5]

Later (in 1899) Daniels (*see* above), who was based in British Guiana between 1896 and 1898, concluded:

> The differences observed both in the male and female are sufficient, I consider, to differentiate this from the other described adult filariae. The name '*Filaria Ozzardi*' might be retained for the new species.[6]

Therefore, when Low was researching in the West Indies, doubt remained on the correct designation of the organism(s) originally found in St Lucia and British Guiana: *F nocturna* was already well accepted (*see* above). Was he in fact dealing with one or two under-researched helminths of man? There was also doubt as to whether or not the *new* specie or species caused significant pathological consequences in humans.

Reference and Notes

1   G C Cook. *Disease in the Merchant Navy: a history of the Seamen's Hospital Society.* Oxford: Radcliffe Publishing 2007: 630.

2   (Sir) John George Craggs (1856–1928) was a chartered accountant, and a Member of Council of the Institute of Chartered Accountants. From 1897 until 1906 he was also Hon Secretary of King Edward's Hospital Fund. His publications included works on the voluntary hospitals. He was knighted in 1903. [*See also*: Anonymous. Craggs, Sir John (George). *Who Was Who 1916–1928.* London: A & C Black 5th ed. 1992: 184.]

3   Seamen's Hospital Society; The London School of Tropical Medicine. 'A short account of "The Craggs Prize", from 1899 to 1911'. Presented at a meeting at the Mansion House, presided over by the Rt Hon The Lord Mayor, Wednesday, 28 February, 1912: 4.

4   P Manson. On certain new species of nematode haematozoa occurring in America. *Br med J* 1897; ii: 1837–38. [*See also*: G C Cook. Charles Wilberforce Daniels, FRCP (1862–1927): underrated pioneer of tropical medicine. *Acta Trop* 2002; 81: 237–50; D I Grove. *A History of Human Helminthology.* Wallingford, Oxon: CAB International 1990: 734–6.]

5   O Galgey. *Filaria demarquayii* [sic] in St Lucia, West Indies. *Br med J* 1899; i: 145–6. [*See also*: *Op cit*. Note 4 above (Grove).]

6   C W Daniels. The probable parental form of the sharp-tailed filaria found in the blood of aboriginals of British Guiana. *Br med J* 1899; i: 1459–60. [*See also*: *Op cit*. Note 4 above (Grove).]

Chapter 3

The Caribbean in the late nineteenth century: a contemporary account

An almost contemporary account with that of Low's expedition of some first impressions of the Caribbean (including the disease pattern) has been given by a member of the first MCC[1] tour of the West Indies in 1895; the Captain was a Middlesex amateur – R S Lucas. Barratt's (he was a Norfolk player) account largely relates to cricket, but descriptions of local scenes and customs are of interest:

28 January [1895]:

> I wake up just as we are entering the harbour of Bridgetown, Barbados [see Figure 3.1 and Chapter 5]. We anchor about a mile from land, all amongst the fleet which is quartered here. The ship is surrounded by blacks who sell fruit and dive in a most wonderful way for coins. Also a native band come in a boat and make a fearful row. An inspector comes to see the ship's papers and to see if there is any sickness on board. Also a deputation arrive to welcome the cricketers. We part with our recent friends and steam for shore, where several thousand people thronged the landing place and cheered us. We are taken in private carriages and driven to our hotel where a most delicious breakfast was provided. In afternoon we went to practice. Quite a thousand people came to see us, goodnatured simple niggers but with keen appreciation of the good points of cricket. I hear first three days we have to go to 3 dances, tonight one given by General Leech the commander of forces. The hospitality of the people is unbounded. The strangeness and beauty of the place is unlike anything I have seen before. Everything is provided for us free of charge. They evidently wanted us to win.

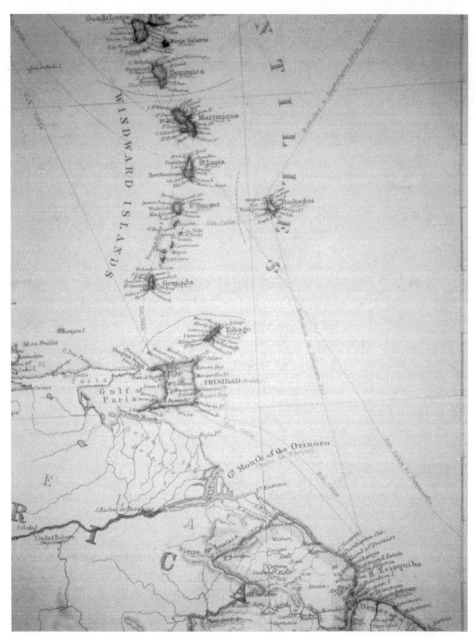

Figure 3.1: Contemporary map of the West Indies, including the Windward Islands –
where Low was to carry out researches during his possession of a Craggs Scholarship.
Courtesy of the Royal Geographical Society (reproduced with permission). [*See also*:
C A Bayly (ed). *Atlas of the British Empire*. London: The Hamlyn Publishing Group Ltd:
1989: 40–5; Anonymous. *Philip's Atlas of the World*. London: Octopus Publishing Group
Ltd; 2006: 321–3; Anonymous. *The Times Comprehensive Atlas of the World* 12th ed.
London: Times Books: 2007: 114 and 116.]

11 February:

> We leave Barbados. A number of people come to see us off. Quite a touching parting. We all sing Auld Lang Syne.
>
> A very charming mountainous island [this presumably refers to St Lucia – *see* below]. A great change from the flatness of Barbados. We stay here about 2 hours in which time I send off a parcel and letter. Journeying on a placid sea we arrive in Martinique at 1 o'clock. This is the most beautiful island I have yet seen. Arriving at Dominica in the afternoon, touching the beautiful town of Roseau ...

13 February:

> Very early in the morning at Montserrat. Continue our voyage in rather a choppy sea to Antigua. The water changes from a deep blue colour to emerald green. We pass the wreck of the Strathyre, which went down in striking the diamond reef in 1891. Hardly anyone was saved. Part of the hull, the funnel and masts are clearly visible. A deputation meet us as we anchor in the harbour and take us to shore in a launch during awful heat. The harbour here is swarming with sharks. A few hundreds meet us on the wharf and we drive to the hotel. A large tennis party was given in the afternoon by the Chief Justice ...

16 February:

> We sail at 7pm for St Kitts [*see* Chapter 9], which is 60 miles away. In leaving Antigua I must say I was not agreeably impressed with the hotel & town – the houses are inferior, the food not so well cooked, the shops inadequate & a general air of slovenliness. They are much more independent & not nearly so civil. We arrive at St Kitts at 12.30 midnight & even at this time we are met by deputation on board ship, rowed a mile to shore in the moonlight where we are surprised to find a large crowd awaiting our arrival. We are taken to the club & have drinks, then on to the hotel & into bed, which we are very ready for.

17 February:

> We go and see the cricket ground in the morning. It is quite the most picturesque ground I have ever seen – situated high

above the town of Basse Terre it commands an extensive view of the harbour & bay of St Kitts & is surrounded on one side by steep rugged mountains. … After lunch we went for a 10-mile drive into the country to see a place called Brimstone Hill, a fortification occupied by English soldiers until 1814. It is a very hard climb up to the top & we only managed to get there through the aid of divers drinks. At the foot of this peak is a leper asylum on the edge of the sea. We went to see them. There were 68 **lepers** there all suffering from that horrible curse, some having no hands, some no feet. Even under these circumstances they seem fairly happy & sing hymns most beautifully. We send them some of our old cricket bats. We drive home in the cool of the evening.

20 February:

Leave St Kitts. Finest climate of any island we visited, beautiful harbour, very rich in cultivation of sugar & cocoa. Very fine scenery & a very pleasant contrast to Antigua in the buildings & general tone of the place.

21 February:

We are steaming along all night, passing Montserrat in the early dawn, too early for me to catch a view of the island. Between Montserrat & Dominica we view a vessel flying the distress flag so have to leave our course & go & help her. We find she is a Brazilian steamboat, her machinery having gone wrong. She was in danger of drifting onto the rocks. We turn her head around & set her going the other way & are all promised salvage money. Arrive at the beautiful town of Roseau, Dominica about 2 pm where 14 ponies have been ordered to meet us & we all ride through what is believed to be the most wild & beautiful scenery in West Indies. It seemed so to me. We rode through deep gullies & dark ravines, at times on the very unprotected edge of some vast abyss, through forests of limes, the humming-birds all round us. The air was filled with beautiful odours. We arrived at the summit, having a bird's-eye view of the broad Atlantic. Returning we see the glorious effect of the setting sun on the mountains, too lovely to describe. We have a delicious drink of lime squash & a cigarette with the

Royal Mail agent & return to the 'Esk' en route to St Lucia via Martinique. We arrive at St Pierre at 10.30 in evening. 4 of us go ashore for an hour. Most amusing experiences. The dress of the Martinique girls is very charming & is world-famed. They are all of French extraction.

22 February:

Arrive St Lucia [then a British Colony – *see* Chapters 4 and 8] 6 am. Usual deputation meet us & hand us one or two invitations. Stop at Gov. House – Governor away on leave ...[2]

The following description of the history of St Lucia is based on an account by Morris:

Southwards from St Lucia are St Vincent and the Grenadines (*see* Chapter 7), and to the east side lies the Atlantic, and to the west the Caribbean. It is a volcanic island, the twin peaks being called the Pitons; the centre is mountainous. St Lucia's history had been stormy; it had been involved in the Napoleonic wars, and had passed from France to Britain, and Britain to France 14 times, depending on which power had gained the supremacy of the West Indies. Although it was finally won by the British in 1814, in 1897 it apparently remained 'Frenchified' and the population (mostly negro or mulatto) spoke a patois of 'antique French and rustic English'. The laws and cooking were partly French, and many of the place names were (and remain) French: Trois Grand Point, Vieux Fort, etc. The capital town was, and is still, called Castries after an eighteenth century French Minister of Marine. In 1897, the elite of the island consisted of a small landed gentry of creoles.

The population of St Lucia was 47,000 in 1897; at least 40,000 of them were negroes or mulattoes, and 3,000 to 4,000 creoles (who owned the plantations). There were also 2,000 Indians (imported as labourers for the sugar plantations) and about 200 British (mostly merchants and Civil Servants) – the 'rulers' of St Lucia. Relations between whites and negroes had not been entirely happy since the emancipation of the slave – which had half ruined the planters, who remained embittered (*see* below). It thus possessed a very different atmosphere from the very *English* island of Barbados!

The official community was centred around Government House. A mile or so from here lies a plateau above Castries – the Morne (*see*

Chapters 4 and 8). Here a monument marked the spot where Sir John Moore [1761–1809] had stormed and captured Fort Charlotte in 1796. It was on the Morne that a huge bonfire had been lit to celebrate Queen Victoria's Diamond Jubilee in 1897. The island was both a military and naval base, and on the Morne was a rambling yellow barracks – built on an Indian design. The soldiers were not encouraged to go sea-bathing for fear of catching malaria! In a trough around the Morne, guns embedded in stone, and ammunition bunkers burrowed in the hill behind – guarded the harbour entrance. St Lucia is one of the finest natural harbours in the world and was, at the height of the Empire, an important Imperial Coaling Station; in 1897, 15 Royal Navy ships called at Castries every month, and during that year, 947 ships entered Castries – 620 of them steamships; in tonnage handled, Castries was at that time, the fourteenth most important port in the world.

The island's English newspaper was the *Voice of St Lucia* (*see* Chapter 5, and Letters XI, XXVI, and XXVIII), whose editor in 1897 was R G McHugh, according to Morris, 'a very argumentative man'.[3]

Barratt then continued his narrative:

23 February:

> Finish match v St Lucia. … After the match we go up to the garrison above the town on a mountain 2000ft called the Morne [*see* above and Chapter 8]. It commands a beautiful view of the harbour & its guns can cover any ship that enters. … Officers are a capital lot & we are very sorry to leave St Lucia on the next day.

24 February:

> We leave St Lucia by special boat, the Weir, very small and uncomfortable. St Lucia is undoubtedly one of the most beautiful islands but the town is far from beautiful, being very dirty and abounding in bad smells from inadequate drainage systems. We hear afterwards that whilst we were at the barracks there was a case of **yellow fever** [*see* Chapter 8] up there which was kept dark. A month afterwards 2 or 3 more cases were disclosed. St Lucia is very useful to England as a coaling station. We leave the wharf at 8 am & sail through a very rough sea to St Vincent [*see* Chapter 7]. … Met by members

of committee who take us for a picnic on horseback to a place they call the Soufrière that is a sulphur lake 3500ft from sea level. This is one of the show places of the world. We commence our ascent into the clouds. I, coming rather late, get hold of a very bad pony. It was very welcome to get under the shade of a tree & have cold oranges fresh picked off the tree & drink iced whisky & soda. In 2 hours arrive at the top, where we see a huge extinct volcano, not having been in eruption since 1812, when the lava was then thrown as far as Barbados 90 miles away. It was quite dark in Bridgetown with falling cinders. The present dust in Barbados is attributed to this eruption. Very giddy looking over this vast precipice. We return with some difficulty as it is so steep that the horses can hardly help stumbling. We row to the ship & continue our journey to Kingstown, St Vincent. We lie and sleep on the deck until our arrival at 10 o'clock. Large crowd receives us. I am quartered with 3 others at the club.

26 February:

Start by RMS Esk 8.30, steam through some charming scenery, arriving at Grenada [see Chapter 7] at 5 o'clock pm. Grenada is a very pretty cocoa-growing island with one of the very best land-locked harbours. At the wharf we find a masquerade is going on. Everyone wears a charming mask. Wonderful sight in the marketplace – great fight there. We drive to cricket ground, which seems to be wedged in between two precipitous cliffs. … St George is the name of the town & is a charming spot …

27 February:

Our much looked forward to arrival at Trinidad [see Chapter 7] takes place the next morning at 6 o'clock. We passed the Bocas rocks just at daybreak. It is here very like Scotch loch scenery. A large deputation came on board to receive us – amongst them Capt. Cust ADC Mr Knollys Colonial Sec. Sir John Goldsby – the Solicitor-General & about 20 others. Driven first to the club (which is the best yet seen in West Indies) here we all have cocktails & egg swizzles*, then on to the hotel which is

---

*Brandy cocktail.

a fine building on the edge of the Savannah (almost exactly corresponds to our Common). After more cocktails about 100 sit down to breakfast …

2 March:

Eventful day. I start from Gov. House at 8.30 & drive a gentleman's tandem 10 miles through most beautiful scenery passing through several coolie villages & in passing cannot help noticing the scantiness of their clothing & the multitude of their jewelry, each coolie girl having as a rule 4 or 5 bangles on each wrist. They also have rings through their noses and silver rings on their toes and ankles. They each represent a jeweller's shop, as anything they wear is for sale. The Blue Basin is a beautiful crystal pool at the foot of a waterfall. Here we first have swizzles & then sit down to a very nice breakfast. We dismiss the ladies out of sight & bathe in the round clear pool; after dressing again, the ladies return very cautiously peeping round the rocks to see it all is right. After lunch we all go to the Gymkhana race meeting. I rode in a race & jolly nearly got killed. Mr Bush also had a fall & being very heavy he got a nasty bruise. One of the niggers got hold of his leg & tried to pull him off.

6 March:

Beautiful swimming bath we have in the gardens here. Most of us visit it once a day. It is about 50ft long & 8 or 10ft deep & the water is almost too cold early in the morning. … Dance in the evening of about 150 people. Admiral Meade is a thorough American. In talking to him of his ship the 'New York' he says 'she has everything that any other man-of-war had & a bit more besides I guess'. I enjoyed the dance immensely. Some very interesting American ladies there. The lancers & polka were danced in the American fashion, which was indeed curious.

13 March:

Early this morning the mail from England arrives. Our morning is spent in packing. Farewell is the order, & it is with feeling of regret that we drive away from this beautiful residence where we have spent such a very good time. I look back on our visit here as the brightest of many very bright experiences. Another affecting farewell took place onboard the Dutch steamer 'Prince Wilhelm' and at about 9 pm we steamed away from South America. We had not been long on the 'Prince Wilhelm' before we discovered she was an exceedingly dirty & uncomfortable boat & I must say that I spent 2 days on this boat which I shall not readily forget.

25 March:

I hear the report of the cannon fired as the mail boat from England anchors in Bridgetown [Barbados] harbour. It was a very welcome sound to me as it heralded the approach of the mail letters from England. Sewell & I rowed before breakfast across to the mail boat which was the 'Atrato' & had a cocktail on board. She is a fine ship, with beautiful hurricane deck. I looked at her with some interest as I knew that we should spend more than 3 weeks on her as she was to take us to Jamaica & back to England.

Our voyage to Jamaica was of the pleasantest description. The voyage lasted 4 days. We passed the isle of Hayti [sic] during the 3rd day. Hayti is very interesting as it is one of the few black republics, with a president. A white or even coloured man is not allowed to own or even to occupy any land there. In fact no alien to a Haytian is allowed to remain there. I was told that it was impossible for a President to remain so long unless he disposes of all his enemies, either by poison or by shooting them. An Englishman lands here at his own risk. I have heard many tales of how white men have been robbed & sometimes murdered there. A favourite trick they have, when they come with an idea of robbing you, they oil themselves all over & come quite naked, so that they are too slippery to catch hold of. In the interior of the island they are still cannibals, being especially fond of babies.

29 March:

At 6 am in the morning we find ourselves anchored in Kingston harbour, Jamaica. I see the American fleet are here & find out afterwards they are waiting here so that at a moment's notice they can slip down to Cuba 90 miles – where a rather serious revolution is impending. Cuba belongs to Spain & the Cubans want to cast off the Spanish yoke & have a republic similar to Hayti …

31 March:

We drove 6 miles to Constant Spring Hotel situated just at the foot of the mountains. … We continued our way through the most exquisite scenery, ever ascending until about midday we arrive at Castleton, one of the showplaces of Jamaica. The gardens are full of all kinds of rare exotics, plants, fern, orchids. We have lunch at a little hotel – mountain mullet, ring-tailed pigeon. Lighting our cigars, we drove home in the cool of the afternoon & as it was downhill all the way the light American buggies rattled along at a rare pace.

2 April:

The Myrtle Bank Hotel, though very large, is far from comfortable. The food is exceedingly tough & unpalatable & the number of flies which infests the dining saloon is enough to turn one from one's food.

We found today a *scorpion* on one of our cricket bags. I got it put into a bottle which I still retain. The sting of this reptile is very venomous.

On arrival at Myrtle Bank the previous Friday a man who inhabited the next room to me was suffering from **typhoid fever**. I felt quite an interest in him (although I had never seen him) as he used to keep me awake all night vomiting & groaning. He was removed from the hotel on the Sunday & was dead & buried on the Tuesday.

4 April:

We catch the 8 o'clock train from Kingston. Had some ham sandwiches & claret en route. Some of the views from this railway have been considered to rival any scenery in the world. The journey was unbearably hot & I was not sorry when we caught sight of the deep blue sea & descended from the mountains to Montego Bay, where we were to stay the next two days & play a match v W. Jamaica …

6 April:

> ... In the evening we attended a banquet. I had the pleasure
> of sitting at dinner next the black bowler Lewis who was the
> ugliest black man I think I have ever seen. He however talked
> very intelligently to me during the whole time & afterwards he
> was called upon & made a very good speech. Knibb, another
> black, also spoke. The usual toasts followed & we finished by
> all joining hands & singing 'Auld Lang Syne', the everlasting
> band still being in attendance.

7 April:

> An eventful day. Not very sorry to leave Montego Bay. The
> food & accommodation were of a very primitive nature. The
> *mosquitoes* were more ravenous & also venomous than any
> place I have yet visited & I had no protection from them in the
> shape of a mosquito curtain. (*After four hours in the buggies*) we
> arrive at a place called Falmouth at 11 o'clock.
>
> In the programme it was arranged that we were to lunch at
> Mr Sewell's who owns the finest estate in Jamaica. The drivers
> of our buggies said they had orders from their master not to
> go out of their way to Mr Sewell's. Consequently when we got
> to the fork road which turned off to Mr Sewell's it was evident
> that there would be a row as we were determined to fulfil our
> engagement. The drivers proceeded to take their horses out
> in direct disobedience to our orders. A fracas ensued which
> might have ended seriously as they use their knives out here
> with very little provocation. Our driver was easily persuaded
> to put his horses in again, but several of them had to be for-
> cibly taken by the scruff of the neck & compelled to do so. One
> of the onlookers got his knife out but soon put it back again.
> When the drivers found they were getting the worse of it they
> consented to go. Barker got a little scratched by one of them.
>
> We arrived at Mr Sewell's about 1.30. It is quite the most
> beautifully situated house I have ever seen, standing as it does
> 1500ft immediately above the sea, the different estates lying
> like a map below. Sitting next to Mr Houchen at lunch I had a
> long talk about Norfolk & several mutual acquaintances. I am
> afraid I had indulged a little too much in the old rum as I slept

calmly & peacefully for several miles, which is not an easy matter with 3 in a buggy. The distance from Mr Sewell's to St Ann's Bay was 27 miles – up hill and down dale. I thought our ponies would never last the 66 miles as they looked so thin, but they struggled on & brought us safely to our destination at St Ann's Bay at about 9pm. A beautiful hot dinner was waiting for us.

8 April:

Most of us went to bathe at a place called the Roaring River Falls or Elfin's Grotto. This is by far the most picturesque place (how odious comparisons are) which I have ever seen in the W. Indies.

We are all put up at a private house. The bedrooms have been turned into dormitories. We are all aware this evening, from divers bites & itchings, that we have become associated somewhat closely with that abominable insect the *Jamaica tick*. It is a little insect, almost always caught from the grass. It bites very sharply & is very difficult to get rid of.

10 April:

We start from St Ann's Bay on our drive to Ewarton, where we are to catch the train back to Kingston. Driving through one village we met a black woman running towards us with a white baby, which she seemed very proud of. As we passed, she shouted Look! Look at my white baby! There is nothing they are more proud of than this, I am told. After traversing miles we come to the celebrated Fern Gully. Lord Hawke,[4] a man who has travelled all over the world & seen everything, said this was the finest sight in the world.

It was exceedingly hot. Fortunately just before reaching the summit we met a boy carrying a can of fresh milk, which we very quickly shared amongst us. Although we had enjoyed our stay in the country very much & had seen many wonderful sights well worth seeing, still I was not sorry to get back to Kingston & have a fixed place of abode for a few days & also to get rid of the ticks, of which we had all got a fresh supply in the Fern Gully.

12 April GOOD FRIDAY:

> Five of the team, Lucas, Priestley, Barker, Wakefield & myself,
> had a most enjoyable excursion to a place called Newcastle,
> where a division of the Leicestershire Regt is stationed.
> Newcastle is 4200ft immediately above the sea. A vast precipice
> is always on one side of the path. Several places were pointed
> out where soldiers had fallen over & one where a lady had been
> precipitated from her pony's back right over the precipice. But
> our steeds were as sure-footed & more so than human beings
> & carried us safely to the top. It had the reputation of being the
> most dreary & lonely place in the world where British troops
> are quartered. Even with that glorious view, watching the
> mails come & go to England & no doubt ever dreaming of the
> time when the mail will take them to return no more.

13 April:

> … In the evening Priestley & I went to dinner with Sir Henry
> Blake,[5] Governor of Jamaica. Julian Hawthorn (the American
> author) & his wife were there. I had the honour of taking in
> Miss Blake to dinner, who was a very nice girl with good looks.
> She intimated that she was going to England on the 'Atrato'.
> Priestley got entangled in an argument with Lady Blake on the
> Home Rule question. Lady Blake is an Irish woman & conse-
> quently held very strong opinions on the subject which did not
> coincide with those of Priestley. However with divers nudges
> & winks I managed to get him away.

15 April:

> This the last day of our visit to Jamaica was spent by almost
> all the team in the morning preparing for our departure on the
> following day, changing Jamaica money into English money,
> drawing cheques for the passage home & buying cigars and
> curiosities. We all went by the 1 o'clock train to the Jamaica
> races. Looking at the racecourse, one might have imagined it
> to be an English one, with the green sward & white railed-in
> course – but the tall waving palm trees, gigantic banyans & the
> multitude of excited black faces soon dispelled these notions.
> The interest in horse-racing in Jamaica is stronger than in any

other sport, and almost every man of wealth owns one or two racehorses.

The Governor's box was especially reserved but Sir Henry Blake [*see* above] did not appear. Lady Blake told me that the last time they attended the meeting there was a dreadful row, ending in a free fight with sticks; several of the more excited blacks collecting outside the Governor's box & threatening him. We could quite imagine this happening from the frequent fights which occurred almost after every race.

After the last race we caught the special train back to Kingston & after a hurried change & a still more hurried dinner, we drove off to our farewell dance at the Constant Spring Hotel. We saw many of our Jamaica friends for the last time & I was exceedingly sorry not to be able to participate in all the parting cups which my friends wished to take with me – if I had done so I am afraid I should have been left among the dead men under the table …

16 April:

The day of our departure from Jamaica has arrived with all its packings, rushings about, card leaving & farewells. The black boy Barnes who has acted as valet to me during my stay in Jamaica gave me his card & offered to come then or at any date as a servant to me in England – he was a very good boy & if I had been placed in a position of wanting such a youth, I would gladly have taken him … .[6]

References and Notes

1 Marylebone Cricket Club (MCC) – which at that time dominated the cricketing world.
2 I Barratt. The first Caribbean caper. *Wisden Cricket Monthly* 1994; 15 (no 10): 20–21, (no 11): 46–47, (no 12): 48–49; 16 (no 1): 36–37, (no 2): 36–37.
3 J Morris. *Pax Britannica: II: the climax of an empire*. London: The Folio Society 1992: 408.
4 **Martin Bladen Hawke** (1860–1938) had succeeded his father and became the 7th Baron in 1887. He was educated at Eton and Magdalene College, Cambridge and became a well known cricketer and captain of Yorkshire (1883–1910). He was later President of MCC (1914–18). [*See also*: Anonymous. Hawke, 7th Baron, Martin Bladen Hawke. *Who Was Who, 1929–1940*. London: A & C Black 2nd ed. 1967: 608.]

5 **Sir Henry Arthur Blake** GCMG (1840–1918) was Captain-General and Governor-in-Chief of Jamaica from 1889 until 1897. He had previously served in the Bahamas (1884–87), Newfoundland (1887–88), and Queensland (1888–89). He was later Governor of Hong-Kong (1897–1903) and Ceylon (1903–07). [*See also*: *Who Was Who, 1916–1928*. London: A & C Black 5th ed. 1992: 76].

6 *Op cit*. See Note 2 above.

Chapter 4

Introduction to the West Indies: filariasis and malaria in St Lucia and Dominica (January–May 1901)

Having obtained the Craggs Scholarship from the LSTM, Low elected to spend a year or two in the West Indies – focusing on the Windward Islands. He sailed from England in late December 1900, arriving at St Lucia in early January 1901. During the first four months there he was introduced to 'medicine in the tropics', and to 'tropical life'. He explored the islands both from an entomological and helminthic viewpoint and also a natural history one. However, as his correspondence with Patrick Manson (1844–1922) (*see* Figure 4.1), which began on 12 January 1901 indicates, he over-emphasised the possible *clinical* importance of *Filaria demarquayi* (now re-named *Mansonella ozzardi*). Low's other major interest here was to document the **malaria** situation in the Windward Islands; there were no previous reports which could be regarded as accurate. He later encountered an outbreak of **yellow fever** (*see* Chapter 8).

A base at St Lucia

Low initially made his base in St Lucia (*see* Figure 4.2 and Chapters 2 and 3) and from there he travelled to several of the Windward Islands and British Guiana (now Guyana). At the time of Low's stay at St Lucia, the long-serving British inhabitants of the island were apparently somewhat disillusioned with the state of the Empire; following the abolition of slavery (in 1833), the adoption of free trade, and collapse of the sugar market they had been left 'high and dry'! But the island still retained important functions as a British naval and military base, and a coaling station.[1]

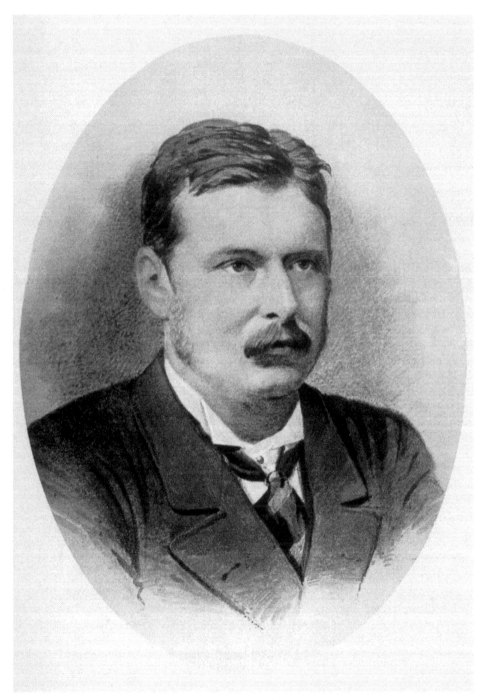

Figure 4.1: Dr (later Sir) Patrick Manson FRS, GCMG (1844–1922) with whom Low corresponded throughout his Caribbean tour.

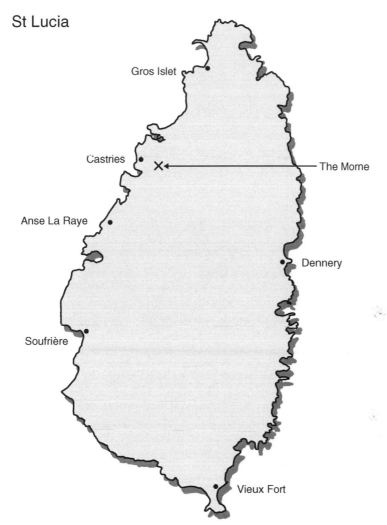

Figure 4.2: Map of St Lucia showing locations at which Low worked. [*See also*: J Morris. *Pax Britannica*: *II the climax of an empire*. London: The Folio Society: 1992: 408.]

Research in the Caribbean

Low was to spend a great deal of the next few months working on those forms of filariases endemic to the Caribbean islands. Clearly Manson's wealth of experience, and also his own interest, in this field formed the motivating force. Some years later, he was to write about *Filaria demarquayi* which was to occupy a great deal of time during this expedition:

... [this organism had been] discovered by [Sir] Patrick Manson in blood slides sent to him from the West Indies, from St. Lucia and St. Vincent by Dr. Otho Galgey[2] and Dr. C. Newsome[3] respectively, and he had given the above name in honour of Jean Nicholas Demarquay (1814–75) who first discovered the embryos. On arriving at St. Lucia, ... Galgey informed me that the slides he had sent ... Manson were taken from one village of St. Lucia – Gros Islet [*see* Figure 4.2] by name, and that he believed most of the cases of this parasite were to be found there. Accordingly I investigated the subject and found that the belief, with one possible exception, was perfectly correct, the parasite was limited to this one village of the island. St Lucia had one main town Castries [*see* Figures 4.3 and 4.4] and five subsidiary townships or villages – namely, Soufrière, Vieux-Fort, Dennery, Gros Islet and Anse-la-Raye [*see* Figure 4.2]. On examining the blood of people from these different villages I got the following results. ...[4]

Low proceeded to carefully document results he had obtained on positive blood slides in different parts of St Lucia, and also in the other Caribbean islands he was to visit during the subsequent 15 months. He often used abbreviations in these letters; however, the major *mosquitoes* (which he often misspelt) he encountered were: *Culex fatigens, C taeniatus, Anopheles albipes* and *Aëdes aegypti (= Stegomyia = C fasciata)*.

With great industry and enormous energy, he travelled between, and worked at St Lucia, Barbados, St Vincent, Trinidad, Grenada, St Kitts and British Guiana (Demerara).

Soon after his arrival at Castries, Low's correspondence with Manson began.

Letter I

Post Office
Castries
St Lucia
Jan. 12th. 01

Dear Dr. Manson,
The mail I believe does not go till the 22nd but I shall begin this letter to night and finish just before it is time for it to leave.

I arrived here safely. We had two terrible days after leaving England, getting into a regular gale which seemed to culminate in the Bay of Biscay. I spent the first two days in bed, though I got up for a little the 2nd day to look at the sea. After that things improved and we got into better and warmer weather. No one appeared at meals at first but after a day or two they gradually began to improve in health and we were soon nearly at full strength.

After I got known a number of people began to ask me about the **malaria** experiments[5] and took a great interest in me when they knew I was coming to the West Indies. I met some important people on their way out to the various islands, and impressed on them as much as possible the *mosquito* malaria infection. I think a lot of them will adopt netting for their windows, and if not they will certainly sleep under *mosquito* nets.

My fellow cabin passenger was a Jamaica planter and he introduced me to a number of men, the Colonial Secretary of Jamaica a Mr. Oliver, and the Chief Justice of Antigua being amongst them. Mr Oliver was a man of few words but he drank [sic] in the facts I think. I met a Dr. Hutson of Barbados and got some good information from him, especially on **filarial infection** based on clinical facts. In an office in Barbados [where the ship first called] was a man heavily infected with filariae, his clerk a white man became infected, after that 4 different clerks all white men coming from families with no filaria all developed the disease. All these men slept at their own homes. Besides this very evident case he said that many white people got the disease in Barbados, in fact that it was by no means uncommon. On the way from Barbados to St. Lucia I was again lucky meeting Dr. Nicholls[6] of Dominica the **yaws** man Dr. Gray[7] of St. Lucia and a Mr. Watts government chemist of Antigua. … Nicholls was very keen that I should pay a visit to Dominica, and as there are Caribs[8] there I said I would. The Chief Justice of Antigua also suggested a visit to that island and I said I would try if possible to pay it a visit.

I arrived at St. Lucia and have put up at a boarding house where Gray, whose wife is at present at Barbados is staying. I called on Dr. Dennehy[9] the Colonial Surgeon next day and also on Dr. Galgey.[10] The former is elderly and knows nothing about microscopic work but is very nice and hearty. Dr. Galgey I am not sure of, he thinks he knows a lot about **filarial diseases** but I

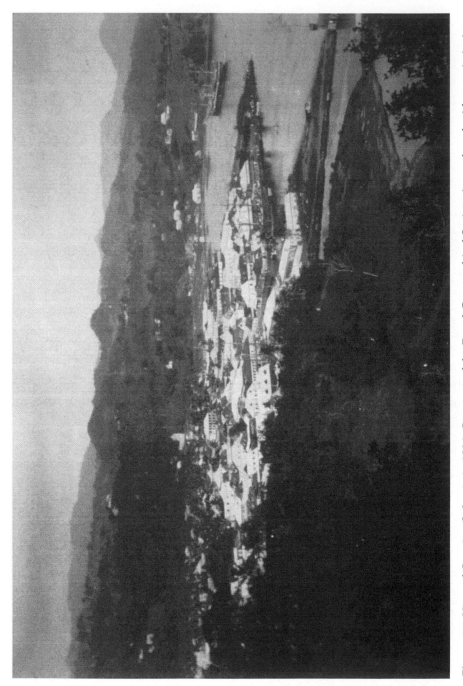

Figure 4.3: View of Castries, St Lucia in 1896. Courtesy of the Royal Geographical Society (reproduced with permission).

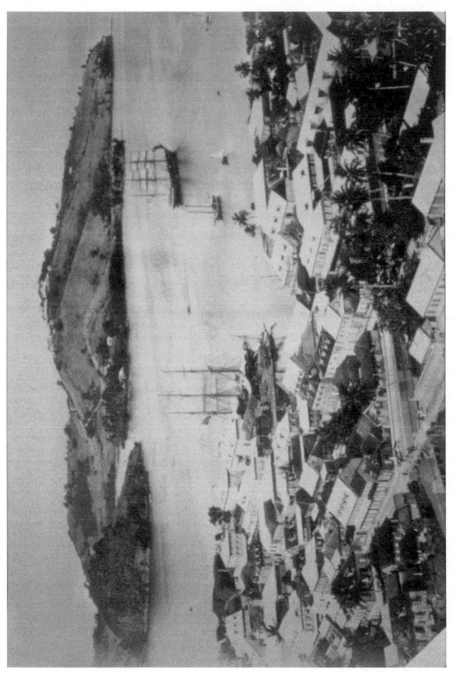

Figure 4.4: View of St Lucia harbour in 1896. Courtesy of the Royal Geographical Society (reproduced with permission).

don't know if I shall get much help from him, but did not seem very keen when I suggested examination of the hospital people at night. He thought the natives would object to have their blood examined. I may of course have judged him wrongly. However I am exceedingly careful not to offend anyone. The 3rd. man is Gray [*see* above], a man after my heart who is very keen on microscopic work and who in the short time I have been here has shewn me things and helped me in no end of ways. Besides those there are the military Doctors, one an especially nice man who is going to let me examine the people in the military hospital. I called on the administrator at once, from what he said he had not received information from the Colonial Office yet, but I hope their letters will arrive next mail.

I was asked and went to a large At Home at Government House last Friday evening. The naval and military officers were in force. These are the chief social points of interest, now for work.

I got begun the 3rd day taking the people in the boarding house for a start. I found to my satisfaction or rather I should say the opposite, that Mrs. Myers the owners of the place, a servant, and a little white french girl all have *filaria nocturna* embryos[11] in their blood. I luckily had ordered a *mosquito* net the first night before I knew this and since then I have taken good care that it fits accurately and that there are no holes in it. So far I have not found *F. Demarquaii*[12] [sic] in the town. I believe it is generally found in the country.

I am trying to buy a pony and then I start for the country districts in earnest. So far my programme is, Examination of the blood of the people in Castries, then statistics of *F. Demarquaii* [sic] in the country where [I have] found prevalence &c then I shall procure a boy suffering from it, take him on as a second servant and try the various insects on him. If I find it is not got in the town it will probably be a country insect, an *anopheles* perhaps, that is responsible. The distances are much greater than I expected and the time will be longer than I thought, but I am not wasting more time that I can help. Already I have gone with Gray [*see* above] to the **yaws** hospital and this morning I took my microscope to the dispensary and examined bloods of people there for him all morning. The result was a poor case of *F. Demarquaii* [sic] from the country and 5 malignant malarias [*Plasmodium falciparum*] the blood in all showing any amount of parasites. Two were in babies with no definite symptoms. I saw a malignant parasite[13] sporulate in the peripheral blood which was lucky. From these observations it is evident that there is plenty of **malarial fever** about though I have not yet seen *anopheles*. To morrow I go with Gray [*see* above] to Soufrière [*see* Figure 4.2] a village down the coast in a coasting steamer. Though it is very hot I am enjoying the life very much and intend to make this my headquarters for some months as there is a fine field for good work.

I hope you are keeping well. The worst of this place there are no newspapers and only a few meagre telegrams so one does not hear much of what is going on in the outer world. I hope you had a good time after I left down in the country and that Mrs. Manson and all the rest of your family are well.

With best regards
Believe me
Yours sincerely
G. C. Low.

P.S.
I enclose some stamps for Miss Manson.

G.L.

Jan. 17. 01.
The mail goes to morrow so I shall close up with a few lines.

Things go on well. I went with Gray [*see* above] to a village Soufrière the other night and got 30 bloods. So far 3 have [F] *Demarquaii* [sic] tho few. I go down again to morrow. I did not think at first that we would get many but luckily I suggested the Police Office. They thought it was a bit of a joke and got quite a number of people in. The slides ran short but I said I would come back again and I expect many will turn up there. Took the Police Force here last night 30 slides.

I have just bought a pony to day and I shall now start to do the country thoroughly. Riding is the only way one can get about. I went the other day with Gray [*see* above] to the dispensary a second time and again got 5 malignant malarias [*P. falciparum*]. One child had no symptoms but wasting. Blood contained – Crescents, ring forms, pigmented leucocytes and marked irregularity in size and shape of corpuscles. Spleen big. There is evidently plenty [of] fever about.

I must stop now but will write you next mail to let you know how things go on.

Believe me
Yrs. &c.
G. C. Low

Letter II

Post Office
Castries
St Lucia
Jan. 30. 01.

Dear Dr. Manson,

Things have gone fairly well since I last wrote you. I have now examined over 300 peoples' blood. I find in Castries itself there is a fair amount of *F. nocturna* [*Wuchereria bancrofti*], and cases of *F. Demarquaii* [sic] occur. Most of the *F. Demarquaii* [sic] cases are got at a place called Gros Islet near the north end of the island. This place is flat and surrounded by well marked swamps full of *anopheles* larvae. It is an ordinary native village.

Down towards the other end of the island I had a try at another village at the mouth of a valley surrounded by hills except where the river breaks through. Here there are large stagnant swamps and plenty [of] *anopheles*, but in this case out of about 30 people examined none had *F. Demarquaii* [sic]. The next place lower down I found 3 cases of [*F*] *Demarquaii* [sic] but little [*F*] *Nocturna*.

I suspect one of the *anopheles* found in the island is probably the host. I have got larvae from the different places and am now breeding from them, waiting now for a suitable case to get bitten e.g. preferably a boy with plenty [of] embryos in his blood. Dr. Galgey [*see* Letter I] says he is to try and get a case but he is rather slow in his movements and I am looking out for one as well myself. **Filarial disease** is now very prevalent [but] not nearly so bad as Barbados for example. As I say I have done 300 examinations but I want to get more if possible. I have not done the hospital yet, they seem to make such a fuss about it. I expect to do it some of those days. I put all odd time by doing malarial work at the Dispensary here. I think of writing a small paper with Gray [*see* Letter I] on the *mosquitos* and **malaria** of St. Lucia. We have collected a good number of facts. I have visited most parts of the island which are inhabited. There is much more **malarial fever** than I thought. The people here are all very kind. Galgey [*see* Letter I] is to be all right I think but as I said before he is rather slow in his movements and does not seem to value time as I do. All the people get more or less lazy out here. The military doctors are nice men and I shall get a lot of the West Indian troops to examine later. I shall make this my base for taking some of the other islands but shall not leave here for some time yet for that.

There has been a quiet time after the Queens death,[14] but really with the exception of mail day nothing goes on here.

I shall stop now.

With best regards to yourself and Mrs. Manson.

Believe me.

Yours sincerely

G. C. Low

Letter III

Castries

Feb. 12. 01.

Dear Dr. Manson,

Excuse this paper as I have run out of more. I send home this mail a piece of tumour from the back of a mans hand suffering from the disease which is called **Pian Cayenne**.[15] I think perhaps it will interest you. The disease is got in wood cutters in Cayenne [French Guiana]. It seems to start from a local inoculation and in the developed state one sees a number of granulomatous masses on the part affected. The nearest thing I can think of it resembles, being a local tuberculosis as seen in Butchers. The disease as I said before is got in Cayenne. It is not **yaws** Gray [*see* Letter I] tells me. It is evidently a definite disease of its own due to some inoculable virus. The case came to dispensary here one day. He had got infected in Cayenne. The back of the hand and lower arm were covered with those tubercles, just over the wrist there was a large mass evidently from many being grown together. Round this were smaller and isolated ones. The surface of said tubercles were smooth reddish no crust or pus and on pricking blood came out. Gray [*see* Letter I] very kindly cut one of the smaller tubercles, which I have preserved in alcohol and send home to you in order that you may have sections cut of it.

I have been making a collection of *mosquitos* but it will not be ready by to morrow. I was to have sent some ankylostoma also but they have not got them for me yet at the hospital.

Work goes on slower than I could wish. I had a man with *F. Demarquaii* [sic] the other night in here and made two *anopheles* bite him. He was a poor case having only one per slide and on dissecting the *mosquito* found nothing. Galgay [sic] [*see* Letter I] was to get me a better case but the boy he sent had nothing at all in his blood. I went to Gros Islet [*see* Figure 4.2] with him yesterday to try to pick up a good case. We saw a man Claude, you will remember the name well as you had slides of his blood in London. I got him to promise to come in to me to night but so far he has not appeared. He is fairly good 5 or 6 to the slide. If I can only get him properly in hand I think he may do, but the people are such a set of scoundrels here that one is never sure of them. I would rather get a boy. I have also got *mosquitos* from Gros Islet to dissect. The disease is not very prevalent in the Island but Gros Islet is the place most cases come from. It is on flat ground at sea level with fine swamps and any amount of *mosquitos, anopheles* and *culex*. An interesting fact is that the people on the heights around don't seem to have it and this makes me more than ever think an *anopheles* is responsible for it. There is not much **malaria** on the heights which also corresponds. I find the *anopheles* here are not house frequenters by day like *Claviges* in Italy. They must live in the woods because though looking carefully for them in houses I have never seen them. They evidently then come and bite people by night. Another point is they are very difficult to keep in captivity dying in a few days, I think that will be got over by trying different foods for them. They bite very readily out of tubes. I have been getting more *nocturna* cases but it is not so prevalent here as in the other islands. I shall infect a series of *culex* now on one of the cases.

Malaria is taking on an epidemic form at present and cases are dying of pernicious symptoms every now & again. I have done 100 examinations for **malaria** taking patients at the dispensary, and out of those there are over 50 infected. That is examining fever cases and children indiscriminantly. Most of the cases are malignant [*P falciparum*] and I have found crescents in 7. Some are mixed infections, and many shew traces of chronic affection with many pigmented leucocytes. This is said to be the worst time for fever and I can quite definitely say that there is plenty in Castries just now. I examined all the cases fresh on the spot. I mean fresh films and I think that is the best way. I am glad to say the administrator asked me to come and see him to talk about the **malarial fever**, to see if anything could be done for it. I suggested several methods and he is to see how far he can carry them out so that is satisfactory. The natives live in huts are ignorant and stupid so one can not hope much for protecting them. If Europeans would only all sleep under properly fitting *mosquito* nets they would escape almost entirely,[16] Then as regards the *mosquito*, I have located plenty breeding grounds quite close to the places where the fever cases are coming from. It is those that I hope to have destroyed because they are small dirty ditches and pools. I think by a good application of kerosene and drainage at small expense the fever of Castries could be greatly reduced. I am to give the administrator a note of the places and I think he will do what is required. I have gathered enough information for a fairly good paper on **malaria** in Castries and I proposed to Gray [*see* Letter I] who has been doing some of the work with me that we should write it together. I shall try and do that as soon as possible now.

I have not got enough for anything on Filaria yet except its prevalence in districts affected &c but if I could only get the host of our friend [*F*] *Demarquaii* [sic] I could have a paper on that also. As I said before I don't get work done so quickly as I would like, but people here don't understand what working at high pressure means and take things very easily. The main thing however is I am very good friends with everyone, and though perhaps slower than I wish they all mean well and shew me things and help me.

I dined at Government House last night and all the officers stationed here have been very kind in asking me out, so with the work I like and some very nice people I have been having a very good time here.

Just to shew you what scoundrels the natives are. I had a very useful boy and was training him to assist at microscope work, and he was shewing marked ability. My silver however used to disappear rather rapidly so one fine morning I caught my friend with 2/= of mine in his pocket. I sent for his grand-mother with whom he lived to come round and questioned her closely to see if she was implicated, but eventually I decided she knew nothing of it. I did not want to prosecute him so I said if she refunded the money stolen I would dismiss only, but at the same [time] I suggested he should be flogged. The old lady jumped at the idea with great alacrity, thanked me for my kindness in words somewhat like these. 'God bless you Sir, God bless you. I shall kill the scoundrel; can you lend me a cane.' I obliged, the renegade was taken down to the yard, in a twinkling of an eye a stool appeared, superfluous garments were removed, and justice administered before a large and appreciative audience of servants and others interested. It shews how difficult it is to try any black man. They steal and lie like anything. I have got another boy, but I think I shall keep him more to look after my pony and to go messages than to come about my room. I have just been examining slides again from the man Claude this morning. They don't shew many filariae so again I must look out for a better case.

I hope you are all well at Queen Anne Street.[17]

With best regards to Mrs. Manson and yourself & family.

Believe me
Yours sincerely
G. C. Low

P.S. I hope the tumour arrives safely. I think it is packed securely. Sections of it will be interesting. You might tell Rees.[18] I shall write to him and try and get ankylostomes for him. Ask him to write me saying what he wants.

G.C.L.

Letter IV

Post Office
Castries
Feb. 27. 01

Dear Dr. Manson,

I had hoped to be able to give you the pleasant tidings of the intermediary host of *F. Demarquaii* [sic] this mail but alas my hopes are doomed to disappointment. I fed *Anopheles albipes* and *Culex*

Taeniatus on a case of Dr. Galgay's [sic] [*see* Letter I] at the hospital the other day. In the only *C. Taeniatus* that bit, 30 hours after feeding I found 26 embryos living and apparently healthy in the blood in the stomach. I thought this looked promising so fed more. However after the blood in the stomach was digested the embryos also totally disappeared. I just dissected 4 this morning. In one at 50 hours after feeding I found some dead & degenerated worms in some of the same digested blood that remained in the stomach. In the other 3 the blood had all gone and in those there was not a ghost of a worm in the muscle, malphigian tubes, or any other portion of the *mosquito*. The conclusions therefore are that *Anopheles albipes* and *C. Taeniatus* do not act as hosts. The next *mosquito* I shall therefore take up is *C. Fatigans*. I have not got any but shall start collecting larvae to morrow. I got your letter last mail and was very glad to hear from you. Before I got it I had been more or less just doing what you advised. I have been doing the different *mosquitos* for *F. nocturna* also. I think I may summarise the results briefly.

Anopheles albipes – 8 infected on a case of *F. Demarquaii* [sic]: result nil. *C. Taeniatus* 6 infected. 30 hours after, in blood in stomach 26 living embryos in one insect. Other 5 examined 50 hours after – result absolutely nil. Special attention paid to malphigian tubes.

For *F. nocturna.*

Culex Fatigans 1 examined. Young embryo in thoracic muscles – *Culex Taeniatus*. I have been doing a series of this, dissecting one daily and find that this insect acts as an efficient host. I have traced them up to the sausage stage with commencement of mouth, alimentary canal &c. I believe there is no *C. pipiens* here. Gray [*see* Letter I] tells me in those sent home [to] Austen & Theobald[19] say it is *C. Fatigans*. As **filariasis** is endemic here it therefore follows that they must act as efficient hosts. As I say I have got advanced forms in *C. Taeniatus* and have seen young forms in the muscles of *C. Fatigans*. I have got to do the series of the latter to definitely make sure of it.

I still think a *mosquito* must spread [F] *Demarquaii* [sic] and though disappointed at not getting it at first it has only whetted my appetite to find it all the more. I know all the *mosquitos* that are found in the island and shall go through them seriatim. If I fail in that I shall go on to fleas, bugs, and other insects. I take a great interest in dissecting and studying the *nocturna* embryos in the *mosquito*, especially after having sectioned them. I find it easy and if I could only hit the right insect would soon get at the [F] *Demarquaii* [sic]. I am making collections of infected *nocturna* insects at the same time in weak alcohol, and will soon be able to send you specimens home if you like. I have not found a case of mixed infection yet, nor a case that I can say is very heavily infected. I infected my insects on an old woman of Dr. Galgay's [sic] [*see* Letter I] at the hospital; average 26 to the slide, still that is good enough because the *nocturna* insects were infected on my servant. 16 to the slide and in some I got as many as 5 or 6 developing in the thoracic muscles. The old woman is a perfect terror, as suspicious as a fox. The last time I had her bitten she yelled moaned & howled all the time. I have not relaxed my efforts to try and get a boy as a servant with [F] *Demarquaii* [sic] embryos. I could then have a good grip of him and examine him hourly. One point of interest I have noted is the [F] *Demarquay* [sic] embryos have a cephalic armature. I have seen the small spine protruding but am not certain if there is [a] prepuce. I could not see a V spot but as the embryo was moving a little I could not be certain. These points I shall look into in detail.

Elephantiasis is fairly common. In 3 cases so far examined no embryos. I saw a good case of Lymph scrotum & chylocele the other day. Strangely enough I could only get 3 embryos to the slide. My only wish is that I could get on faster but things move slowly in the tropics.

I have got notes from Gray [*see* Letter I] of another case of **Pian Cayenne** [*see* Letter III] which I think will interest you. It seems to be a more advanced case than the one I told you about. (By the way I hope you got the tumour). In the man I saw, as I said the disease seemed to start from a local point of inoculation. He had the tubercles on the back of the wrist and of the left hand and also a few on his elbow but nowhere else. From Gray's case it would seem then than [sic] if untreated it may spread pretty well over the whole body. It is not **Yaws** however being quite different. There were no signs of ulceration in the case I saw, but it seems if it lasts long enough that this may take place.

I was very sorry to hear that our report [*see* Letter I] was not yet in at the Colonial Office. I hope by now it is, but if not you might press the matter with Sambon[20] as it is exceedingly slack. I see the other malarial reports are in. The Colonial Office must be wondering why on earth ours is not. The C. Office have written very nice letters about me I believe. I had a letter from Surgeon General Lovell[21] from Trinidad offering to help me in every way when I get there and to get cases ready.

I hope you keep well. I hear the weather at home is very cold. I could spare you some of our heat nicely. It is a beautiful island this, covered with all sorts of tropical vegetation. I got a very fine snake the other day, a non poisonous one. I keep him in my room. There are no parrots or monkeys here and very few birds. I have not had time to examine birds yet, though I have done several dogs. I think I told you it was very hilly so one does ones moving about on horseback.

The negro is a lazy dull headed creature and I have a good lot of trouble getting [co-operation]. I was interested [in] Prout's [22] paper. It is a pity the blood was not examined oftener. I must stop now as it is time for the mail. Hoping to have better news next time.

Believe me.

Yours sincerely

G. C. Low.

Letter V

Post Office

Castries

St. Lucia

March 14. 01

Dear Dr. Manson,

I have a good lot to write to you about this mail.

Firstly in connection with Dr. Gray [see Letter I] I have told you already that he is a very able man who is practically lost in a place like this. He has heard from the treasurer of Sierra Leone who was passing through here that there are likely to be 2 vacancies for a Colonial Surgeon on the West Coast of Africa soon. He would like to go in for one of those to better his financial position and to have a better scope for work. He has a wife and 3 children, and if by chance he got one of those posts he would keep them at home to educate them seeing them when he had leave. At present he is here with no prospect of a rise and even though he got on here the money is not very much. He would fill the post of Colonial Surgeon any where with satisfaction as he is up to date in his work and is a very good operator. Since I have been here, he has done 2 hysterectomies, the abdominal operation, and both have done well, in other smaller operations he is also good and what is more to the point up to date in his antiseptics. In microscopic work he is also good and if he had more time would go in for it more. I think he is going to write you this mail also. If you can do anything to help him for an appointment for the West Coast as Colonial Surgeon when a vacancy arises I should be very pleased, and I don't think you would be disappointed in him.

Nextly I send you home by this mail tissues from a case of **elephantiasis**. A woman had her leg amputated for this to day, and I had a good dissection of the limb afterwards. Left foot and lower part of leg affected. Amputation through knee joint. On dissection I got a gland (enlarged) from the popliteal space and the lymphatic[s] leading into it. I could not find any dilatations of the lymphatics in any other part. I have taken a smear from the gland and also from the lymph[sic] in different parts of the leg to examine for ova or embryos. I cannot examine those to night as there is no light but shall do them in the morning and will put in the result. I thought the best thing was to send the gland home and you can have it sectioned and perhaps it may shew something of interest in elucidating the pathology of the disease. In the same bottle are [a] piece of skin & pieces of subcutaneous tissue a nerve and a piece of vein. The leg presented the usual appearance of hypertrophy of the skin and subcutaneous tissue, the muscles were flabby and a lot of lymph exuded from every part. No hypertrophy of the bone or of the blood vessels. Examination of the blood before operation no filaria.

I also send you in a different bottle a tumour from the ear of a native – I think just an ordinary fibroid. These 2 bottles I have sent to your house. I have also sent a box of *mosquitos* to Rees [*see* Letter III] at the school. They are of interest and you might get them classified. There are specimens of *Culex Taeniatus, Anopheles albipes,* 2 species of a brown *mosquito* one larger than the other; the smaller of the 2 is *Culex fatigans*. The larger you might get Theobald [*see* Letter IV] to name. There are also 2 very minute *mosquitos* I think of a genus quite different. I think they are new. They are very small black in colour, hind torsi white with a peculiar proboscis. They may only be a small species of *culex* but I think they are probably different. I think the 2 brown *mosquitos* are undoubtedly different. I want specially the name of the big one as I am going at him for the *filaria Demarquaii* [sic].

Now about *F. Demarquaii* [sic]. Anatomy of fresh specimens. Head has a cephalic armature there is a prepuce not as distinctly seen as in *Nocturna* and as far as I can make out not serrated. ... This prepuce one can see drawn back every now and then disclosing a spine very much resembling that of *Nocturna* and very minute. There is a V spot again not so distinct as in *Nocturna* and more obtuse as to its angle. I don't think one need fear the *taeniatus* as a spreader of the disease and just as well as they are in millions here. Before to morrow afternoon I shall have dissected a lot more and will let you know the result.

What do you think I should do now? Do you think I should stay on here pursuing the host of *F. Demarquaii* [sic] or sh. I get on to Demerara [British Guiana] and trust to find it there. Of course the work I have done here is very useful and facts though negative are always of importance. One does not see much of the Pathological effects of *nocturna* disease here though plenty of the people have embryos in their blood. With the exception of Gray [*see* Letter I] one does not gain anything from the Doctors here; Galgay [sic] [*see* Letter 1] although thinking he knows a lot about filarial disease is really perfectly incompetent in microscopic [work], and for the matter of that in any other work besides. He has not a record of a single case and never knows if such and [such] a man has embryos in his blood or not.

Dennchy [*see* Letter I] the Colonial Surgeon laughs at the whole thing and thinks it is a fiasco; he treats his fever cases with calomel and worm powders. This of course is bet. ourselves. I am quite friendly with all of them, and take care not to offend them though one cant help laughing at their old fashioned ideas. I hope for Grays sake he will get a better appointment because as I have already told you he is a really good man. I am in communication with Nicholls [*see* Letter I] of Dominica, Newsam [*see* above] St. Vincent and Hutson of Barbados all of whom are wishing me very much to appear at their respective islands.

Whenever you get this letter write me and say what you advise; that will be about a month before I get your answer. I think myself I had better be moving on to some place where there is more disease. Amongst other things working at the Dispensary with Gray [*see* Letter I] I have examined 215 cases for **malaria** and though I have not my figures added up have got I think over 100 infected. About 18 cases of crescents. We have been trying to infect *anopheles*, but have run out of stock at present. In one that died a few hours after feeding we saw zygotes but will have to have more to see how far they develop. If we could get this done we will write a conjoined paper on **malaria** in St. Lucia. If you like I could write a short paper on some of the intermediate hosts of *F. Nocturna* or perhaps I should wait till I do some more in the other islands. Say what you think? I hope all the sections I sent have arrived home safely.

The weather is beginning to get very hot now and I have to sit with precious little on when working. I explored a part of the interior of the island one day. It was very interesting but very hard work. One had to cut ones way through an impenetrable virgin forest with a cutlass. One of the officers here and myself went. We walked up a river bed for 3 miles or so which was lined with dense forests wh. met in a canopy overhead making it quite dark. From there we clambered up a ravine with hands and feet and then cut our way up to the top of a mountain through all sorts of tropical vegetation. Results from a scientific view disappointing. I got the *mosquitos* I told you of before on the top, a small specie of *culex* wh. bit freely. I saw only 2 birds and no snakes. Unfortunately in whacking a tree with the cutlass I cut a very fine spider in two. We got our hands badly cut and both of us fell several times on the boulders of the river bed. I shall get right across the island next week to a village I have not been at yet. I hope to strike some **filaria cases** there. There are a lot of very nice officers here, as St. Lucia is now an important military station. More troops I believe are coming. The military doctors are both very nice men and let me go to their hospital when I like. I must stop for to day now but will finish to morrow before the mail. I enclose some stamps for Miss Manson.

Friday noon.
I have just dissected 18 *culex taeniatus* 17½ days after feeding. All except 2 show no filariae and the positive ones shew each 2 filariae that have undergone no development at all.

The conclusion is that though filariae go to the muscle and develop in an irregular & poor manner they eventually are gradually absorbed and disappear. This eliminates *taeniatus* as a host.

I must stop as it is near the time for the mail to close.

With best regards to Mrs. Manson and the rest of your family.

Believe me

Yours sincerely

G. C. Low

Letter VI

Castries

March 27. 01

Dear Dr. Manson,

Again I have to report failure as regards finding the intermediate host of *F. Demarquaii* [sic]. I have just the small large brown *mosquito* specimens of which I sent you home and find they are quite blank. The small and large brown *mosquitos* are however I am now sure, the same *mosquito*, the fact of some being larger than the others depending on age or favourable food. This brown mosquito is according to Theobald [*see* letter IV] (e.g. in a letter to Grey [sic] *Culex fatigans*). According to that there is no *pipiens* here at all. Of *C. fatigans* more anon in its relation *to F. nocturna*. You might however get Rees [*see* Letter III] to have the specimen I sent home identified so as to make perfectly sure. In last letter I told you of finding a sausage stage in a *C. Taeniatus* that had fed on a case *F. Demarq.* and said I thought it must be a *nocturna* embryo. How the contamination occurred I cannot say but there is no doubt it was one. To satisfy my mind I started all over again and bred out more *taeniatus* and then fed them on a good case of *F.D.* In every instance the result was absolutely negative. I find that as long as there is blood in the stomach of a *C. Taeniatus* or *C. fatigans*, one can see *Demarquaii* [sic] embryos there, but as soon as the blood goes they also disappear meaning that that species is not an efficient host and that they are gradually digested. Measuring such embryos there is no increase of size and one can gradually see that the cells of the body degenerate. I always of course examine every piece of the whole body of the insect brain, ovaries, Malphigian tubes &c.

The *mosquitos* were fed on different cases with *Demarquaii* [sic] embryos and the patients blood was always examined at the same time to see that the embryos were there. However, I am certain they are not hosts because it was always easy to see embryos swimming in the blood of the stomach but whenever that went, they also went.

I also have dissected *mosquitos* of similar species caught in the bedrooms of people suffering from the diseases, likewise with negative results. This cuts out the 3 common *mosquitos* of the place *Anopheles albipes*, *C. Taeniatus* and *C. Fatigans*. Of other *mosquitoes* I caught a small species of *culex* in the bush one day miles from any human habitation in the depth of the virgin forest. This is the only place one finds it so it cant be a host. I once saw a small black *culex* in water from a ditch but I have never been able to find it again. There are some other genera, *aedes* [sic] &c which don't bite. I wonder if fleas, lice, or bugs can spread it. I shall try and get every insect I can lay hands on and shall start and see if I can't find some other species of mosquito.

Nocturna experiments [author's italics]:

The efficient host for this parasite is *Culex Fatigans* at which I am working now. At 4½ days after feeding the filariae are at the large sausage stage. At 5½ days dissected this morning, thorax full of filariae changed now from sausage stage and become elongated. Mouth, alimentary canal and anus beautifully seen. If the rate of development goes on as quick as it is going, (which I shall see in the next few days) they will reach maturity in about 10 days I sh. think. That however one will have to see.

Though the embryos go to the muscles of *C. Taeniatus* I don't think it will prove to be an efficient host as Rees [*see* Letter III] found in the sections he did in London. Few after 5 days are seen developing in the muscles. At 7¾ days they are at the large sausage stage. At dates after that they develop further but not in the same definite way as in *C. Fatigans*. I found one large one, one day. I am doing a batch at 17½ days after feeding now. 2 dissected this morning had nothing: one a degenerated form of a fairly developed form and another had 3 small forms that had not developed at all.

The development therefore is irregular & feeble. I have plenty waiting to dissect and shall see if they ever get to the proboscis.

I can't see a tail spot. There are nuclei in the central body cavity and those are enclosed by a striated musculo-cutaneous layer. The embryos locomote freely through the blood pushing their way with vigour right through masses of corpuscles. Another feature is they often attach themselves by their head to the cover and then their body moves about while the head is fixed. They may keep like this for a good time ... I suppose this is what Grassi[23] describes for *F. Recondita*.

Next as to the host I have a very peculiar thing to tell you. Well I had nine *C. Taeniatus* bite a man with *F.D.* the other day. I dissected them 72 hours after feeding. 8 blanks but in one (no 9) I found a well developed sausage stage of a filaria ... in the muscle. It was exactly like the stage of *F. Nocturna*. At once I thought it must be a *Nocturna* but against ... that the man was fed in a new house which had had no ones hand [sic] it [was] before 11 AM in the morning, ie there was no chance of me having left a *mosquito* that had sucked a *nocturna* case in the box. Of course insects reared from larvae.

The next fallacy that came to my mind was could Claude the man also have *nocturna* embryos. Against this was the fact how could you have such a large developed sausage stage in 72 hours. And also that though I had not examined him myself at night for noct. embryos Galgey [*see* Letter I] said he had (though that may not go for much). Also we have had many of the same mans blood slides at home (Claude) and I never saw any noct. embryos. The peculiar thing is if it was a *Demarquaii* [sic] embryo how should none of the other *culex taeniatus* have been infected because most were fed on a woman with far more embryos than Claude. This give[s] rise to the idea could it have been another species of *mosquito*. It certainly to all intents and purposes looked exactly like the other *taeniatus* in the tube. I cant quite explain it but my [sic] the weight of opinion is against *F.D.* embryo. That it was an embryo is certain; it moved and I have now seen so many *nocturna* sausage stages in *culexs'* dissected that I have no doubt as to its genuineness. The thing is uncertain however, so don't say anything about it.

I am hard at work at two species of brown *mosquitos* now, the ones I have sent home in the collection. The worst of them is they wont bite by day so though I tried Claude for 2 hours I failed to get any to bite. He lives 9 miles from town and won't stay the night. I sent a lot up to the hospital today to bite the woman to night and I hope to hear they have been successful in the morning. The worst now is the old woman makes such a rumpus that she has to be held down when the *mosquitoes* are to bite and it is difficult with her wriggling about to give them a chance. I want to get another case but it is no joke getting the people from the country even tho I try heavy bribing. They are a set of suspicious fools. However tho there are difficulties I am pegging at it as hard as I can.

I have been keeping and dissecting many infected with *nocturna* following out the stages. (In *C. Taeniatus*). I have 20 infected which I am carefully keeping to try for proboscis specimens. I shall pickle some when ready to send home.

Friday 15. Just examined smears from gland, and those from lymph [sic] of leg. Nothing to be seen of ova or embryos. I send you a photo (poor print) by Gray of the pigmented areas in an old **yaw** case. I have negatives of the same case & we will get better prints.

The boy has just come back from the hospital. The woman made a tremendous fuss last night I hear and only one *mosquito* got a little blood. The man is to try them again to night. Results will have to wait over there.

I must stop now as the mail is almost closed.

With best regards to Mrs. Manson your family and yourself.

Believe me

Yours sincerely

G. C. Low

Letter VII

Castries

April 10th. 01

Dear Dr. Manson

I send you a short paper by this mail, which I have written on the development of *Filaria Nocturna*. You might read it and see what you think of it, and send it to the *British Medical Journal* [author's italics].[24] You will see that the complete metamorphosis is got at this month of the year in 11 days. I believe it is quite possible in the hot weather to get it at 8 days or 9 days. So I have stated that and uphold your original views. Manifestly temperature is the main feature, which Bancroft[25] did not seem to take into account in his experiments in Queensland. By now you will have had the brown *mosquitoes* I sent home identified. Gray [*see* Letter I] sent similar [ones] to Theobald [*see* Letter IV] who is responsible for the name *C. fatigans*. It is quite easy finding the embryos in the proboscis but it is difficult to say exactly where they lie. I have concluded with a note on the work up to date on *F. Demarquaii* [sic]. It is a blessing *C. Taeniatus* does not spread the disease. The measurements I did very carefully, and there is absolutely no doubt about the variability in length. Change the English if you think fit.

I have been pursuing flies lately to see if they spread *F.D.* Some small sandflies do bite and it is possible they may be the carriers. They are difficult to get and I have had no luck so far in finding anything in them. Whether one can keep them alive in captivity I have not yet had the chance yet. However I set out for another village on Saturday called Vieux Fort [*see* Figure 4.2]. I am to spend 2 nights there and hope to get something. I was over the island last week at a place called Dennery [*see* Figure 4.2]. It was a beautiful ride through the mountains, scenery being perfect. Got a lot of *mosquitoes*, all breeds I had before. I am going to Domenica [sic] on Tuesday for 10 days then back here then will try to reach St. Vincent. Dr. Nicholls [*see* Letter I] has promised to get me plenty [of] blood slides &c. I wonder if I shall find *F. Demarquaii* [sic] in that island.

I had a letter from Rees [*see* Letter III] along with yours last mail. He thinks of going to the Cape I see.[26] We had no rain lately and it is getting fairly hot. One is always getting annoyed by various parasites. The *mosquitoes* are very numerous now, (*taeniatus*) and I have to look very sharply after my net to see they don't get in.

I hope you are all well at Queen Anne Street. Your weather must be getting very pleasant now.

With best regards to Mrs. Manson and yourself.

Believe me
Yours sincerely
G. C. Low

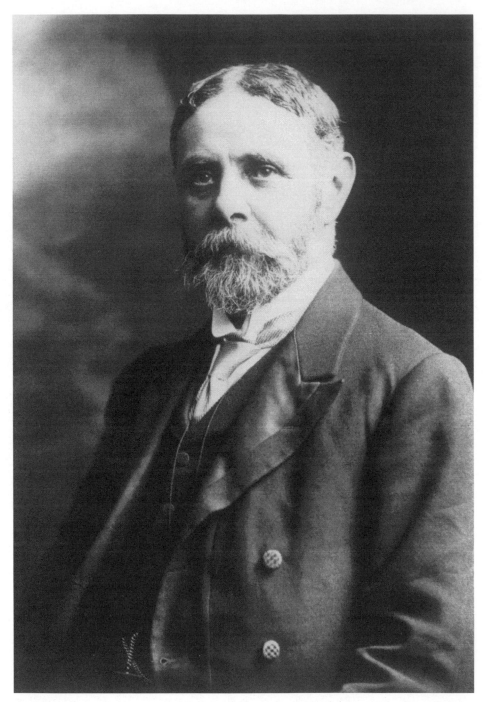

Figure 4.5: Dr C W Daniels FRCP (1862–1927) who was at that time Superintendent of the LSTM. Courtesy of the Wellcome Library, London (reproduced with permission).

Seamen's Hospital Society.

LONDON SCHOOL OF TROPICAL MEDICINE.
ROYAL ALBERT DOCKS, E.

Lectures to Nurses on Tropical Subjects.

Two Courses are given annually at this School, beginning respectively about October 15th and February 15th.

Each Course will consist of 10 Lectures. *including the*

Fee for the Course, £2 2s. ~~Nurses entering for the examination,~~ *examination.* ~~must pay an additional fee of £1 1s.~~ A second examination, if necessary, may be undergone by the Nurse on payment of 10s. 6d.

A Certificate, signed by all the Lecturers, will be given to the successful Candidates.

SYLLABUS.

1. Dr. DUNCAN.	Personal Hygiene in the Tropics, outfit, clothing, exercise, food, alcohol, baths, &c.
2. Dr. DUNCAN.	Enteric Fever and Dysentery.
3. Dr. DUNCAN.	Cholera and Heat Stroke.
4. Mr. CANTLIE.	Abscess of Liver, special surgical requirements in the Tropics, care of instruments, &c.
5. Dr. SANDWITH.	Plague and Beri-Beri.
6. Dr. SANDWITH.	Dengue, Sleeping Sickness, and Blackwater Fever.
7. Dr. McLEOD.	Leprosy, Skin Diseases, Prickly Heat, Boils, Ulcers, Dhobie Itch, &c.
8. Dr. DANIELS.	Malaria and Mosquitoes.
9. Dr. DANIELS.	Yellow Fever, Filariasis, Sprue and Hill Diarrhœa.
10. Dr. LEIPER.	Intestinal Worms, Treatment of Patients preliminary to vermifuges, examination of fæces for the worms, &c.

Further particulars may be obtained on application to the Matron at the Albert Dock Hospital, Connaught Road, Albert Dock, London, E.

2nd April, 1909.

Figure 4.6: Daniels played an enormously important rôle in the early years of the LSTM. He figured prominently, for example, in the list of tropical nursing lectures at the London School of Tropical Medicine (LSTM) in 1909. [*See also*: G C Cook. *Disease in the Merchant Navy: a history of the Seamen's Hospital Society*. Oxford: Radcliffe Publishing; 2007: 630.]

Letter VIII

Castries
St. Lucia
May 1st. 1901.

My dear Dr. Manson,

I was very glad to get your letter of the 12th April and also Dr Daniels[27] [*see* Figures 4.5 and 4.6] about the *mosquitos*. I was especially interested in them and their possible bearing on the *Demarquaii* [sic] business. I was pretty certain when I got the little black one that he was a new genus as he has turned out to be but I don't think he has any thing to do with spreading the filaria as I could not get them to bite and they died the 2nd day after coming out of the pupae. I could not keep them in captivity. I don't think it is likely they bite at all but yet they might in a state of nature. As regards the others the *culices* and the *anopheles* I have excluded them completely. I got a black *mosquito* in the town one day but have never been able to get it again. The ones from the bush cant have anything to do with it as they are never got in the filarial district. They only live in dense bush & virgin forest where no one lives. They bite all right but are very delicate all being dead by the time I got them home. I am determined I shall find the thing but it may take time. I have questioned the people at Gros Islet one of the centres very closely but they say *mosquitos* only bite them. All [those] caught in their houses by them and myself were common and on dissection shewed nothing. One man however told me that when the rains began a fly (wh. I take from his description to be a sand fly) bites them badly. Going on that I dissected some small flies from near an infected house but found nothing; that however means nothing. How to breed and keep sand flies will be a very difficult task. I caught another *culex C. Taeniorhynchus* I think, in a place I have never got **filaria cases** in. It is rare. It is possible I have missed some *mosquito* that spreads it, but the difficulty about the business is that one catches say one of those rarer species only once and then cant [find] them or their larvae again. The dry weather has spoilt everything; all the pools having dried up and the places near where I got those are now no good.

Your idea of it only being spread at certain seasons is I think a likely enough one. Perhaps in the rainy weather. I have been thinking a tremendous lot about the thing and have adopted a new mode of research namely to begin and visit adjacent islands to see if it is got there, to study what places it is found in and to see if any similar insect is got there. By means of this plan I can exclude insects which I cant breed & keep in captivity.

Following out this plan I visited *Dominica* [author's italics], and put in 10 days very stiff work. I am happy to say I found *F. Demarquaii* [sic] in that island is indigenous in people who have never been out it. The place again was on the sea shore at the mouth of a valley like in St. Lucia is on flat ground. *Mosquitos* found the same as in St. Lucia. Now we know it is got in St. Vincent and the point to me now is, is it got in Barbados which is a flat island. The places in St. Lucia are all flat and on the sea shore. I have never found it in people from the mountains. Before I got your letter I had heard there were differences in B. Guiana as to accommodation and facilities for work so I am glad you think I should stick on in this part of the world. I shall go to Barbados as soon as I can get to go on Tuesday the 7th. and shall examine that island thoroughly. I think & hope I shall find it there, and if I do the facilities for work there will be infinitely better [than] this place. They have a large hospital and *filaria Nocturna* is far more prevalent than here. From what I hear they will give me every assistance there. Bet. ourselves Galgay [sic] [*see* Letter I] here is very jealous and that hampers me. I have never even been allowed to examine the hospital patients and have had to do all my work in a little balcony off my bedroom. Again I have had to bribe people to come to the hotel to get their blood the only way possible to get it, in fact do every thing of [sic] my own bat. They have a sort of laboratory in Barbados and I am sure they will let me use it and let me tap the hospital patients. Now that my old friend the microtome has arrived (I have forgotten to mention this so far) I shall be in my element again and start cutting sections of filariated *mosquitoes*.[28] There will be no difficulty getting good subjects to infect from them.

Suppose I do not find *Demarquaii* [sic] in Barbados then St. Vincent is only a 12 hour journey and Dr Newsam [*see* above] has promised to give me every help or I can come back here. My plan then is to go to Barbados to fix up my laboratory there. If *Dem* is found there good, if not I shall go to St. Vincent, get my malarial work as much of it as I can there and take the boat to B. to section. When you write me next address Post Office Barbados.

You have no idea how kind Dr. Nicholls [*see* Letter I] was to me in Dominica. I got a room to work in the hospital and had the free run of the institution and tapped the whole of the inmates of the gaol all the police and many more besides. You will be very interested to hear that I found *F. Demarquaii* [sic] in a case of **elephantiasis** there in Dominica. There were no *nocturna* embryos as the case was somewhat advanced, but it was therefore a case of double infection. I did not get *Dem*. in many cases but still I only wanted to know if it were found in that island. If I had had more time I would have found it in more. I got Dr. Nicholls [*see* above] to amputate an **elephantiasis** leg and again carefully dissected it. I made many smears from the lymph but found no ova or embryos. I have the tissues and will cut them myself now.

Did you find anything in the material I sent home? I have not done as many animals as I would wish here but then there are practically none. There are no crows magpies or jays. You may see a pigeon once in a while in the bush. Dogs I have done as much as possible. I got *immitis* [*see* Letter XI] in one. There is a blackbird about but you are not allowed to shoot them. Bats are present but they are very difficult to get.

I send you by this mail the paper on **malaria** by Gray and myself [*Br med J* 1902; i: 193–4]. I think as no one has written on **malaria** before here it is important that the results are accurate as with only one or two exceptions I did all the blood examinations myself and have verified and send [?] all that is described in it. I shall not bother describing it as you will read it for yourself. The important point is that the W.I. negro differs from his aboriginal ancestor in his susceptibility to **malaria**.[29] I hope you manage to get it into the *BMJ* [author's italics][30] and that it will give Gray a help ... in the chances for his promotion. I suppose you got my little paper on the development of *Filaria nocturna* sent on April the 12th in the different *mosquitoes* here. I hope the *BMJ* [author's italics] have published it. There is nothing much in it except in shewing that *taeniatus* is inefficient, an important point for the West Indies and that temp. is so important a factor, a point wh. Bancroft did not recognise [*see* above].

I think I told you the microtome arrived by the mail. I have thought of what you said about the filariae escaping by the excreta or skin. I don't think myself it is probable but I shall look into the matter. Ticks I have looked at and I have never heard of them biting man, though dogs and cows have plenty. There is no **blackwater fever** in cases here.

I have spent nights in different villages and one of the most awful places was a place called Vieux Fort [*see* Figure 4.2] where I had two nights. To get there one had to get in a little steamer. Only 2 white people live in the place and I had to live in a small police station. The bed was fairly clean but unfortunately they had arrested a lunatic that morning (Saturday) and as there was no steamer till Monday he spent his time almost immediately below my room in a cell. I never heard a man roar and howl like him. I never slept either of the two nights and had to drink polluted river water. Of course I slept under my net and have no doubt that owing to that I got no fever.[31]

Insects were disappointing. I caught some common *mosquitos*. It is supposed to be the worst place for them in the island, but owing to the drought I found very few. I could only by the greatest dint of perseverance get 30 blood exams and strangely enough none had filariae. I went out a whole day and [searched] for insects in the direction where *Demarquaii* [sic] exists and stayed out late at night sitting under a tree but nothing attacked me. The village of Gros Islet [*see* Figure 4.2] where most of the cases came from is exactly similar to all the other villages. It is on flat ground on the sea shore and **malaria** is common as in the rest. It presents no special peculiarity and as I have said the insects seem to be the same. I have searched it carefully but have found no peculiar insect. Perhaps such a host appears in the wet season which will not come for more than a month yet. I am going out that way this afternoon and will again see if I can get any larvae or insects. The weather now is very hot and the sun fairly terrible, our only salvation is the trade wind which blows strong as a rule all day. When it fails the heat is very trying. St. Lucia and Dominica are very hilly and getting about is difficult, everything being done on horseback. I have sold my pony as one can bicycle and drive about in Barbados which is flat. I am looking forward to the insects of that island with special interest. The Doctors and people there say that they have no *anopheles* mosquitos and no **malarial fever**. Now if this is so why should there be no *anopheles*. Antigua is flat like Barbados and has plenty, and also fever. If there are no *anopheles* in B. there must be very definite reasons for it. I expect myself that I shall find them however and fever also, as well as *F. Demarquaii* [sic].

I must send Mr. Michelli[32] a 6 monthly report by this mail to say what I am doing I see it is in the terms of the scholarship.[33] I suppose they will give me it for the following year as I have heard nothing to the contrary.

There is a very pretty parrot in this island but very rare. I have tried to get one to send home to you but have not been able. Monkeys are not found here and the fauna really is very poor.

I think I must stop now as I have exhausted my news. I send the paper under separate cover by same mail. I expect to get to Barbados on the 7th. and will drop you a line by same mail from there.

With best regards to Mrs. Manson your family and yourself,

Believe me

Yours sincerely

G. C. Low

References and Notes

1   J Morris. *Pax Britannica: II The climax of an Empire*. London: The Folio Society 1992: 408.

2   **Otho Galgey** had qualified (LRCSI) in 1871 and obtained the MRCPI in 1886. His research contributions were on filariasis and ankylostomiasis. [*See also*: *Medical Directory*. London: J & A Churchill 1902; 1861.]

3   This possibly refers to **Francis Newsham**, who had qualified (LRCPI, MRCS) from the Royal School Manchester in 1875. [*See also: Medical Directory*. London: J & A Churchill 1909: 830.]

4   G C Low. The unequal distribution of filariasis in the tropics. *Lancet* 1908; i: 279–81.

5   Low's clinical investigations undertaken in the Roman Campagna, had clinched the man-mosquito cycle of *Plasmodium vivax*. [*See also*: P Manson. Experimental proof of the mosquito-malaria theory. *Br med J* 1900; ii: 949–51.]

6   **Hy Alfred Alford Nicholls** CMG was the Medical Officer of Health for Dominica. He had obtained an MD (Aberdeen) in 1875, having qualified MB CM and MRCS in 1873. He had studied at Aberdeen and St Bartholomew's Hospital, and had become an authority on yaws in the West Indies. [*See also*: *Medical Directory*. London: J & A Churchill 1902: 1906.]

7   **St George Gray** was the Assistant (Colonial) Surgeon for St Lucia. He had

qualified from Trinity College Dublin (MB, BCh) in 1887. Currently in charge of the Yaws Hospital at Castries, he had previously been House Physician at the San Francisco Polyclinic. [*See also: Medical Directory.* London: J & A Churchill 1902: 1863.]

8 Refers to the Carib Indians. Members of the native race which occupied the southern islands of the West Indies at their discovery … (J A Simpson, E S C Weiner [eds]. *The Oxford English Dictionary* 2nd ed. Oxford: Clarendon Press 1989; 2: 899.)

9 **Charles Dennehy** FRCS (Edin) was the Colonial Surgeon in St Lucia. He had obtained his fellowship in 1883, having graduated from Dublin (LRCPI & LM) in 1855. [*See also*: *Medical Directory.* London: J & A Churchill 1902: 1850.]

10 Galgey is credited with the first demonstration of adult females of *F demarquayi. Op cit.* See Note 2 above. [*See also*: P Manson. *Br med J* 1900; ii: 949–51.]

11 Microfilariae of *Wuchereria bancrofti* (formerly *Filaria sanguinis hominis*) and named by Manson *Filaria nocturna.*

12 A Castellani, A J Chalmers. *Manual of Tropical Medicine* 3rd ed. London: Baillière Tindall & Cox 1919: 639–40. In 1895, Manson discovered a microfilaria in blood films of 'natives' from St Vincent, which he named *Filaria demarquayi* – after the discoverer . In 1897, he found the same organism in Carib Indians in British Guiana; he initially considered this to be a different species and named it *F. ozzardi.* It is also found in Dominica, Trinidad and St Lucia. The organism is now named *Mansonella ozzardi*; it is not periodic (as is *W bancrofti*), the microfilariae closely resemble *Mansonella perstans*, and it is transmitted (in the Caribbean) by *Culicoides furens* (a midge) and possibly by *C. paraensis* and *C. phlebotomus.* Although most infected people are asymptomatic, joint pains, headaches, coldness of the legs, inguinal lymphadenitis, and itchy erythmatous skin lesions have been associated with a high parasitaemia.

13 Refers to *Plasmodium falciparum*; Low was clearly observing erythrocytic schizogony in a peripheral blood film.

14 Queen Victoria (1819–1901) had died at Osborne House, Isle of Wight on 22 January 1901. She was succeeded by her son (who had been the Prince of Wales for 60 years) King Edward VII (1841–1910).

15 The name suggests yaws; however, the description resembles that of cutaneous leishmaniasis ('pian bois') which had also been documented in Guiana. Cayenne was the capital of French Guiana. [*See also*: A Castellani, A J Chalmers. *Manual of Tropical Medicine* 3rd ed. London: Baillière, Tindall & Cox 1919: 639, 2165.]

16 Advice which has now again come to the forefront of effective strategies for malaria prophylaxis, as no chemoprophylactic or chemotherapeutic agent is now 100% effective.

17 Manson was at that time living at 21 Queen Anne Street, London W1. [*See also*: P H Manson-Bahr, A Alcock. *The life and work of Sir Patrick Manson.*

London: Cassell & Co. 1927: 104–5; G C Cook. Patrick Manson's London residences. *J med Biog* 1997; 5: 186.]

18 **David Charles Rees** (1868–1917) was at that time, the first Superintendent (Medical Tutor) at the London School of Tropical Medicine [Low subsequently became the third Superintendent]. Rees had qualified at Charing Cross Hospital, and was responsible for the School's curriculum – which apparently remained unaltered for many years. [*See also*: Anonymous. David Charles Rees. *Lancet* 1917; ii: 549; P Manson-Bahr. *History of the School of Tropical Medicine in London (1899–1949)*. 1956: 158.]

19 **Frederic Vincent Theobald** FES (1868–1930) was a distinguished entomologist. He graduated from St John's College, Cambridge and, from 1900 to 1903, was in charge of the Economic Zoology Section of the British Museum. Theobald later became Professor of Agricultural Zoology in the University of London. He prepared, for the Colonial Office and the Royal Society, *A Monograph of Mosquitoes of the World* (in five volumes) (1900–11) as well as other learned treatises.

20 **Dr Louis Westenra Sambon** (1865–1931) had accompanied Low on the Roman Campagna expedition in 1900. Born in Milan, he was educated in several countries, qualifying in medicine at St Bartholomew's Medical College and later MD in Naples. Sambon was invited by Manson to accompany Low on the Ugandan sleeping sickness expedition in 1902 (*see* Chapter 1) but could not go, and was replaced by his friend Aldo Castellani (1877–1971). [*See also*: G C Cook. Correspondence from Dr George Carmichael Low to Dr Patrick Manson during the first Ugandan sleeping sickness expedition. *J med Biog* 1993; i: 215–29.]

21 **Sir Francis Henry Lovell** CMG, FRCS (1844–1916) was Surgeon-General and member of the Executive and Legislative Councils of the colonies of Trinidad and Tobago (1893–1901). He was later Dean of the London School of Tropical Medicine. [*See also*: Anonymous. Lovell, Sir Francis Henry. *Who Was Who 1916–1928*. 5th ed. London: A & C Black. 1992: 498.]

22 **William Thomas Prout** CMG was educated at Edinburgh, graduating (MB, CM [Edin]) in 1884. He subsequently spent most of his career either in 'medicine in the tropics' or at the Liverpool School of Tropical Medicine. Prout was a prolific author, focusing on preventive medicine and filariasis. [*See also*: *Medical Directory*. London: J & A Churchill 1902: 878.]

23 **Giovanni Bastista Grassi** (1854–1925) was an eminent Italian malariologist. [*See also*: G C Cook. *Tropical Medicine: an illustrated history of the pioneers*. London: Academic Press 2007: 93–7.]

24 The author has found no evidence that this paper was ever published in the *British Medical Journal*.

25 **Thomas Lane Bancroft** (1860–1933) of Brisbane, Australia, was the son of Joseph Bancroft (1836–94) who had also worked on filariasis. Cobbold (*see* below) had identified the adult worm which had been sent to him by Bancroft senior in 1877; he named it *Filaria bancrofti* in honour of its discoverer; the organism is however, now known as *Wuchereria bancrofti* which corresponds

to Manson's: *Filaria nocturna*. Thomas Spencer Cobbold FRS (1828–86) was the foremost British helminthologist of the nineteenth century. Thomas had sent specimens of *Culex fatigans* to Manson, on which Low had demonstrated *Filaria nocturna* in the proboscis sheath (*Br med J* 1900; i: 1456–7).

26 Rees was about to resign from his position at the London School of Tropical Medicine and emigrate to Port Elizabeth, South Africa, where he died from typhus fever at the age of 49 years.

27 **Charles Wilberforce Daniels** (1862–1927) trained at the London Hospital and qualified MB (Cambridge) in 1886. After service in several tropical countries, including Fiji, British Guiana, West Indies, Malaya, Central Africa and India, he became Superintendent of the LSTM as a successor to D C Rees (*see* Letter III). In 1903, at Manson's request, he became Director of the newly-founded Institute of Medical Research at Kuala Lumpur. It was Manson's intention that the Malayan Institute and the LSTM should interchange personnel and material; however, this failed to materialise. On return to England he became Director of the LSTM, and in 1910 Physician to the Albert Dock Hospital. When Manson retired he became Medical Consultant to the Colonial Office. [*See also*: G C Cook. Charles Wilberforce Daniels FRCP (1862–1927): under-rated pioneer of tropical medicine. *Acta Trop* 2002; 81: 237–50.]

28 Low's initial research project at the London School of Tropical Medicine was demonstration (using the microtome) of the microfilariae of *W. bancrofti* in the proboscis sheath of the mosquito, thus making mosquito to man transmission by the bite of the mosquito virtually certain. [*See also*: G C Low. A recent observation on filaria nocturna in Culex: probable mode of infection of man. *Br med J* 1900; i: 1456–7.]

29 This is an interesting (and topical) theme, but one which Low does not pursue in this correspondence!

30 St. G Gray, G C Low. Malarial fever in St Lucia, WI. *Br med J* 1902; i: 193–4.

31 Avoidance of mosquito-bites was now obviously a very dominant theme in Low's mind; this doubtless arose from his experience gained during the Roman Campagna expedition.

32 **Pietro (later Sir James) Michelli** (1853–1935) was of Italian descent, and served the Seamen's Hospital Society for a total of 57 years; he was the Secretary of both the Society and also the LSTM. He retained the latter position until the London School of Hygiene and Tropical Medicine was founded in 1924. [*See also*: anonymous. Michelli, Sir James. *Who Was Who, 1929–1940.* 2nd ed. London: A & C Black. 1967: 937.]

33 The Craggs Scholarship had been awarded by the London School of Tropical Medicine [*see* Chapter 2].

Chapter 5

Researches in Barbados (May–July 1901)

Having spent four months in St Lucia, Low now sailed to Barbados, principally to study filariasis on that island, and to confirm Manson's Amoy finding in a different geographical setting. Bridgetown, Barbados was his base until he returned to England. He briefly visited several other islands, returning to Castries in late 1901. Correspondence to Manson from Barbados began in May.

Letter IX

Bay Mansion
Barbados.
May 9th. 01.

Dear Dr. Manson,

Just a line to let you know how things are going here. I arrived safely from St. Lucia. Before leaving I made a careful search for insects in the filarial district but owing to every thing being completely dried up there were no larvae to be found of those rare species. Till the rains come there will not be much chance of getting insects.

My reception here was very cordial. [Figure 5.1 shows an almost contemporary view of the capital city – Bridgetown (*see* Figure 3.1) – lying to the south-west of the island]. I have met the doctors and they are to give me every help possible. I have got a room in the hospital and permission to work at the patients there. I have also been allowed to do an almshouse containing 350 people so I should get a tremendous lot of blood examinations. As these institutions have patients from all over the island I shall soon see if *Demarquaii* [sic] is found here. If so I shall get the exact locality. I hope to get 1000 examinations to see its *nocturna* prevalence. Already I have a new *mosquito* which I think I got one example of in St. Lucia. The Doctors are all very keen on the work. **Filarial disease** is called 'fever and

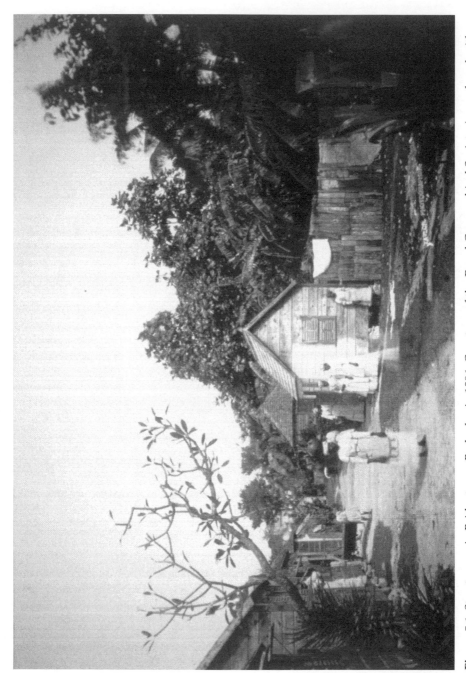

Figure 5.1: Street scene in Bridgetown, Barbados in 1896. Courtesy of the Royal Geographical Society (reproduced with permission).

ague' here and they tell me there is any amount of it about, very common in white people. They say there is no indigenous **malaria** and the point now to be looked into is are there *anopheles*[?]. I tried one very likely looking pool but found only *culex*. I shall do the whole island carefully and shall try to see if any insect or condition exists that should account for there being none. Of course I may find them. I am specially interested to see if *Demarquaii* [sic] is found. If not I shall get a good clue to the host. A man I know goes to St. Vincent on Monday and I am to give him a letter to Dr. Newsam [*see* Chapter 4] to get him to get fleas and other biting insects if possible from infected houses for me and then I shall section them.

I have my apparatus fitted up. The microtome is all right. I have just examined 41 slides from the hospital taken last night and got several slight infections.

I send home some *mosquitos* to Daniels [*see* Letter VIII] in pill boxes and also some ticks. A big consignment of *mosquitos* and flies I shall send next mail and I hope to have some thing interesting to tell you then.

Believe me
Yours sincerely
G. C. Low

Letter X

Bay Mansion
Barbados.
May 24. 01.

My dear Dr. Manson,
Just time for a short line. Things going well. Have examined 500 people here plenty *nocturna* no *Demarquaii* [sic] so far. *Mosquitos* 4 species *fatigans* and *taeniatus*, a small species of *culex* and that new genus with the antennae twice as long as proboscis found in crab holes. I got a P.M. on a *nocturna* case. Man died of sarcoma had not examined peripheral blood as only in 2 days. At P.M. took film from lung found embryos. Proceeded as in your case.[1] Examined 4 specimens from each of the organs and vessels. Lung average 16 to slide, other organs all nil ie. blood films. Slight infection but interesting all being in lungs. Searched for over an hour for adults – did not find them. All [in] the thoracic duct healthy, also pelvic lymphatics.

List of specimens I send home this mail to you addressed to school:-

Box of *mosquitos*. Specimens from Dominica, St. Lucia and Barbados also small flies to see if they are biters and their names.

Particulars written on discs underneath. e.g. the island they come &c. Dr. Daniels [*see* Letter VIII] might get them identified.

2. Box tin with tubes. Tissues from *nocturna* case. Lung &c. 2 pieces of glands, 1 from groin one from pelvis latter looked sarcomatous However [sic] hard venereal probably. N.B. nodule of sarcoma in lung.

2 [sic] Some tissues from a case of **elephantiasis** from Dominica.

3 [sic] Tubes with infected *taeniatus* not of much importance after my fresh dissection of that species but will do for students practising on.

4 [sic] Ticks from Dog.

5 [sic] Larvae & pupae of *C. fatigans*.

6 [sic] Larvae & pupae of crab hole *mosquito*, important for Theobald [*see* Letter IV].

I hope all those arrive safely and in good condition. I have written on each tube the contents. I have kept duplicates to cut here. Interesting to say I have been unable to get *anopheles* larvae in this island though I have searched a very typical swamp and other places.[2] This answers well as the people around it are perfectly healthy and apparently there is no indigenous **malaria**. Why? I am looking into carefully.

Filaria nocturna is abundant. I find no embryos in what is called here 'fever & ague' e.g. Filaria lymphangitis. Some of those are merging into **Elephantiasis**[3] however. I have got through a great lot of work here and am going strong as I wish to get over to St. Vincent soon, after *Demarquaii* [sic] and its host. Still till the rains come there will not be much good going there as every thing is so dry. Interesting no *Demarquaii* [sic] in Barbados so far. You must excuse this very short note as I have been very busy.

The heat is terrible and I feel it pretty trying, however I keep at it.

I hope things go on well at home.

Did you get the malarial paper all right.

With best regards to Mrs. Manson and yourself.

Believe me

Yours sincerely

G. C. Low

Letter XI

June 7 01
Bay Mansion
Barbados.

Dear Dr. Manson,

Things go on slowly tho well. I discovered a new (to me at least) filaria in the tick bird to day. On examining several I came across what seemed like a filaria in peripheral blood taken at 8 A.M. To make sure I killed said bird and got blood from the lungs and heart, and was rewarded by finding any amount. Though spending an hour or so at the body I could not come across the adults. Staining by different methods is interesting. Those with haemalum shew a very long sheath even longer than that of *F. nocturna* tho somewhat similar in nature, both ends of the worm are rounded & it is not easy to say which is the head & the tail! I send you specimens home which you might see if new or not and what its name is. The sheath I think is extremely interesting. I am now to get another infected bird [to] determine if any periodicity exists[4] and try & work out the intermediate host, it might be a *mosquito* or perhaps lice & fleas. Along with the 2 slides which are stained but not yet mounted in balsam I send some *mosquitos* for the school for sectioning. Owing to cockroaches eating through the netting of the house a number of reared infected ones escaped so most of those I send are only from the curtain [sic] of an infected patient being taken, and kept [at] definite times as shewed on labels. One or two may have missed infection and some even may be doubly infected but still they will do for men practising on. I dissected a series of 100 *mosquitos* from 3 wards in the hospital and found 23 infected. Curiously enough all were single infections, in one I got them in the proboscis but as it was ruptured, where they were was difficult to say.

I fear *Demarquaii* [sic] is non existent here as I have now examined 600 odd people from different parts of the island. I get a fair amount of cases of the disease but unfortunately none will die.

The doctors are all very kind to me in getting material and letting me get about the hospital. The Governor [*see* Letter XIII] is responsible for this perhaps as he took the reins in his hands at once and said I was to have every facility and as he is a determined man he means it. This makes things run smoothly and I am getting on with my work.

Though searching carefully I have failed to find *anopheles*. The swamp (there is only one in the island) looks perfectly good for them but I can only find a small *culex* breeding in it, and that *mosquito* I sent home by last mail which breeds in crab holes in the vicinity. The water smells strongly of H$_2$S [hydrogen sulphide] but one sees all sorts of dragon flies and similar insects breeding in it. I shall send you home some of the water to have it analysed. Why other parts of the island are destitute of *anopheles* is simple as there is no water. The surface is more or less flat with a small amount of soil over the underlying coral and when it rains the water percolates through this very quickly. There are several ponds and places I have to examine yet. Rivers don't exist at all, at least not above ground though there must be some very large subterranean ones. Apart from those interesting scientific points it is an uninteresting place, covered chiefly with cane fields. What I am now after is to see if dogs have *F. immitis* [a canine filarial infection] when there so far [are] no *anopheles*. I hope all the specimens and papers I have sent have reached you safely.

I should like a bottle of carbol fuchsin, some xylol, a few little boxes for slides and if you want any large quantities of filariated blood send me one of the big ones and I shall fill it. I think I said I should like some [of] that petit [?] cork for pinning *mosquitos* on. Anything else you would like, let me know. I hope the last consignment of *mosquitos* got home safe as there were some very good ones amongst it.

A Mr. J. A. Martin, a son in law of a Major Bennet here – people who have been very kind to me, is going in for second inspector of Police in Barbados a post generally filled by ex militia officers and of course given by the Colonial Office. He asked me if you would have any influence in the matter at the Colonial Office. I said not being a medical post I did not see how you could but that I would mention the fact to you. If by any chance you could mention his name to Mr. Lucas unofficially in connection with the thing I should be glad but don't put yourself to any bother because I cant see myself that it would do any good as I think the Governor [*see* Letter XIII] here is the man who will decide it. I would have not worried you with this but as I promised the man I thought it better to do so.

I am going to read a paper on **filariasis** to the Natural History Society next week. I have written a short paper putting it as plainly as possible and laying special emphasis on the *mosquitos* there and the prophylaxis. I will shew specimens of *mosquito* larvae &c & it may interest them.

I am delighted after St. Lucia to see everyone taking an interest in these latest researches. I enclose a cutting from the St. Lucia paper [*see* below] to shew you to what a depth of laziness & ignorance they have reached there. Too lazy for any thing. This however is an emanation of the editor of the paper and does not represent the educated class of Castries. I wrote a short report to Sir Harry Thompson the Administrator pointing out how far the fever could very easily be reduced and he took a great interest in this and I have no doubt will act on the suggestions. There is hope for diminishing **filarial infections** here, theoretically there should be none as there is a good pipe water supply from the under ground rivers and reservoirs in the interior and there should therefore be no standing water for *mosquitos* to breed in practically; however tanks for washing, and wells and water barrels for similar purposes still exist and here the *mosquitos* breed & multiply.

A very interesting fact is that in Castries the brown mosquito *fatigans* was about ¼ less numerous than *taeniatus*, while here *taeniatus* is rare [with] *fatigans* predominating tremendously. This accounts for the increased **filarial diseases**. I hope you got my little paper on filaria development [because] I think it is important for this part of the world.

The Governor [*see* Letter XIII] lent me the Liverpool School's report[5] from West Africa. It was very neatly got up pretty pictures &c but not much of importance in it.

By the way what about our report did it ever appear or did it ever go to the Colonial Office[?]. It should have been [as] good as the West African one I think. Liverpool are pushing on evidently and going it. I saw somewhere they had found some new filariae of birds. You had better find out about the one I sent you and if it is new get the credit for London. If you like or if you think my productions [sic] are of any value I could write one [on] **filariasis** in Barbados. Prevalence, conditions favouring its spread, water supply, statistics, percentage of infected *mosquitos* &c. I have plenty of material to go on I think. You might write to me by return to here above address [or] if I have gone I shall be in St. Vincent and they can forward your letter there. If you want such a paper let me know. I think that about exhausts my stock of research news.

Socially this place is all right, there are some very nice people and as I said the Governor [*see* Letter XIII] has been very kind. I dined there one night. There is little to do outside of work, the island is flat and no trees and very few animals on it, no parrots though I believe in one place a few monkeys, the latter being the animals I want to get at. I have made a plan of campaign out for St. Vincent and hope to finish off *Demarquaii* [sic] there. I dont want to stay too long here but wish to finish it off thoroughly. The facilities for work are splendid in Barbados as compared with those other islands so I shall stay on for a bit. I think of going to St. V. for a fortnight first, coming back here and sectioning material &c. The weather is frightfully hot and it [is] difficult getting about in the middle of the day now for the sun. The rains are coming, 5″ falling the other day. I hope Mrs. Manson yourself and family are well.

With best regards to you all
Believe me
Yours sincerely
G. C. Low

Enclosed with this letter (XI) was a newspaper cutting from the *Voice of St Lucia* (undated):

The Mosquito Expert
WE hear, says the *Voice* of St Lucia, that Dr. Low, the *mosquito* expert, has made a report on the malarial and mosquito-producing conditions of this island. The report will, no doubt, add to our stock of scientific knowledge. But, we cannot help thinking that for all practical purposes the bliss of ignorance was in this matter decidedly preferable to the folly of wisdom.

This indicates that by mid-1901, the dangers of disease transmission by *mosquitoes* was still *not* appreciated by most of the lay public.

Letter XII

Bay Mansion
Barbados
June 18. 01.

My dear Dr. Manson.

I was very pleased to get your last letter and to hear that you were pleased with the papers. I have been going as hard as possible since and am getting on well with this island.

I delivered a lecture to the Natural History Society one evening and shewed specimens. This has had a good result, as it has frightened a good lot of people and they are all wanting their blood examined to see if they have filariae. I tried to make the lecture as simple as possible, not to muddle the people as most of them before probably knew nothing about it. Again as there were a good lot of ladies present I cut out almost all the medical parts not to shock them.[6] It has been printed in some of the papers so I send you three which contain the whole lecture. You can read it and see what you think of it. I hope the prophylaxis will make them more careful than before.

What is interesting me very much at present is the lymphangitis cases what they call here 'fever and ague'. As a fact there are hardly any long residents who have not had it and I am trying judiciously to tap as many as I can. The great point in these cases is the disappearance of the embryos [microfilarae] from the peripheral blood. For instance, case of a man 64 had many attacks which 5 years ago no permanent thickening no embryos. Another case many attacks no permanent thickening no embryos last attack 2 years ago. I have records of many more with the same results, some however have permanent thickening and some have gone onto **elephantiasis**. Perhaps the most interesting case is that of Dr Morris the head of the Imperial Agriculture Department. He had his first attack last week and he kindly sent for me and let me examine his blood. He had never had it before the attack was definite and in many specimens of blood I found no embryos. Was his attack then due to the death of the parents and will he if not reinfected get another attack? He is going home in August and I suggested to him to go & see you as I knew you would be very interested in him. Maitland who spoke at the last *B.M.J* [author's italics] meeting about *white people not getting* *filariasis is entirely wrong* [author's italics]; any amount have it here. The Mulatto[7] also is quite as prone as the Negro.[8] The difficulty is getting at the white people to examine their blood as one cant do that without a good lot leading up to it. I must try and get a lot however. If one could only get post mortem examinations, but since the one I told you off [sic] I have never had another. I have not been able to get another bird with filaria which is a great bother as I have a cage full of *mosquitos* waiting to bite such a case. However I shall get a dog in a day or two & hope for better luck. I must do dogs too as so far I have only had a few.

I have been out again to the swamps and now really believe no *anopheles* exist in the island. One of the swamps is a perfectly typical place for them, but I have found none though a species of *culex* breeds there, and many dragon flies. The water smells of H_2S [hydrogen sulphide] but that is all I can see. I am going to get the Professor at the Government Laboratory to have it analysed. There are only three definite swamps, the one I mention is typical, another not typical but in which I got a *culex* (I think *taeniorhynchus*) [from] a creek in the middle of the town, a mango swamp too dirty I believe for anything to live in. Some ponds are found at other parts and these I must [also] see before I shall definitely pronounce on the fact.

I send a box of *mosquitos* again by this mail. I wish it were not so hot as when the sun is up now, it is almost impossible to go out. I shall stop for to day but shall [write] later before the mail goes.

June 21.01
I have not done very much since the day I began my letter to you. I started off at 6 the other morning, rode about 12 miles on a bicycle, and inspected several ponds and other collections of water towards the north of the island. I found nothing in any of them and not managing to get home before the sun was well up felt pretty well done for the rest of the day. The heat and glare was terrible.

I have a good lot of material ready for sectioning and intend to start cutting it to morrow.

I think I shall go to St. Vincent next mail [to] collect material especially *F. Demarquaii* [sic] and bring it back to work up here. I must live again in an infected village and do my best to get that insect. I may say fairly definitely now *F. Demarquaii* [sic] is non existent here as are also *anopheles*. It is a remarkable island in that respect. I think I had better write a short paper to that effect soon now as it is important.

I must stop for this mail as it is just time for posting.

With best regards to Mrs. Manson yourself and family.

Believe me

Yours sincerely

G. C. Low

P.S

I have sent you a box of Barbados *mosquitos* via this mail.

G. L.

Letter XIII

Bay Mansion

Barbados

July 3rd.01.

Dear Dr. Manson,

The time comes round for another mail so I write you a note to let you know of my movements. I have nearly finished Barbados and have written a short paper which I send home to you by this mail, describing the absence of **malaria** and *anopheles*, and some points about the prevalence and prevention of **filarial disease**.[9] I hope you will like it and get it in the *B.M.J.* [author's italics]. There is really nothing new in it, with perhaps [the] exception of the prevalence of **filariasis** amongst the white people. You will read it and see what you think. [?] report on the prevention to the Governor [*see* below] who has taken a great interest in the subject. I think really a lot could be done in the way of prevention.

I have cut some sections lately but it is very difficult for [?] properly out here, it seems to have absorbed water and gets white; however some of the **elephantiasis** sections are very pretty. I would like to get P.M. but they won't come.

My next movements then are, I leave for Demerara[10] on Monday first to go to Georgetown stay a day or two then proceed up into the bush after *Demarquaii* [sic] and *perstans*. The facilities are fairly easy now I believe. I met Dr. Congers [sic] the other day a friend of Daniels [*see* Letter VIII] & he said there would be no difficulty. I hope to live amongst the Indians and to find that intermediate host. I think my plan of going now is best because the weather gets frightfully hot later, and rainy. Even now I expect it will be very rough work and the chances of escaping fever will I fear be slight. However I don't mind the risk.

After a month in B. Guiana I shall come back to Barbados work up my material and then go to St. Vincent and study *Demarquaii* [sic] there again, trying to see if it is the same as the Demerara one & what its intermediate host is. My headquarters will therefore still be in Barbados so when you write still address letters there, as though I may be away when they arrive I shall get them on returning. I fear I shall miss one mail for certain but that cant be helped.

The rains here have begun now and I assure you it comes down in earnest, one night 3″ falling in one hour. Some days it pours all day and one cant get out at all. With the rains the atmosphere is simply saturated with moisture; everything, clothes boots &c get damp and moulds grow on everything in a day or so. Yesterday poured all day, with thunder rattling incessantly. I keep very fit through it all. I weighed myself to day and find I have lost 7 lbs since coming out, I think however it is better losing than gaining weight in the tropics.

From the papers I send you will see that this is a peculiar island ecologically, not a bit like any of the others and also remarkable in having none of those other diseases. I am glad to have had a good look at it. What annoys one is the laziness of the negros and West Indians generally. Though offering 3^D per bird, and 2^D to bleed dogs, I can't get any of those 2 animals. They say they don't want to catch their birds as there are too few in the island, also dogs; as a result I have not been able to get another infected blackbird.

I am going to take my gun to Demerara and intend shooting material out in the bush, parrots and birds of that sort. I expect a similar blackbird will be found there and if not I shall try and get more when I come back. What I want to see is if *mosquitos* spread it or not [?], think of the long sheath, [?] in the haemalum stained specimens. Things here also should [?] in the human line lately and I have not had many cases. I examined Dr. Morris' blood again and confirmed [my] observations that all the embryos had disappeared. I should think his lymphangitis was due to the death of all the parent worms which had evidently been few. I think he is going home in August and I have suggested to him to be sure to go & see you. If one could only get P.M. examination one could clear up a lot on the subject I am sure.

I have taken to bathing in the mornings here, and one day touched what is called a sea egg with my hand.[11] This horrible creature resembles a hedgehog in appearance with enormous bristles sticking out of it. I was unlucky enough to get about 20 of the spines in me and the pain was really very bad. Though the effect passed off in a day one of my fingers is still sore and permanently thickened. I believe however it will eventually get better. My case was not so bad as that of a person who came to bathe one morning; on [?] he trod on the top of one and getting out as quickly as possible he limped away home, and has not been seen since. [?] not again ventured near the bathing place.

I hope all *mosquitos* I sent home arrived safely, I shall get some good material for you at home when in B. Guiana.

As I told you before the governor Sir. F. Hodgson[12] has taken the subject up with energy and intelligence and I think he will make an attempt to get the **filarial disease** diminished in this island. I expect the other Governors in the other places will be equally kind. I am sure the one in Trinidad will as I hear he is very keen on scientific work.

I suppose you are drawing near another B.M. Association[13] meeting again. Where is it to be this year?

They do a good number of operations out here in the hospital and what strikes one is the remarkable recuperative powers of the negro. It is really a fairly healthy place, Barbados. There is some **enteric fever** [typhoid fever], none of the epidemic diseases such as **plague, cholera** &c, no **liver abscesses** and I don't think proper **tropical dysentery**. Ordinary troubles – **tuberculosis, pneumonia** &c are common and of course **filarial diseases** are very common – no **malaria** which is a blessing.

I have no more news of interest but will leave this open till mail day in case anything else happens.

Believe me,

Yours sincerely

G. C. Low

P.S.

July 5. 01.

I have nothing more of interest I fear to tell you except that we have had a storm to day.

As this is the hurricane time of the year one is never sure what is to happen but I don't think perhaps it will come to anything. The wind was very high this morning with ... tremendous rain accompanied with the thunder and lightning. The weather is really very bad now, and yesterday before the storm broke was very oppressive.

I shall write you next from B. Guiana.

I send you the papers in a separate envelope.

Yours sincerely

G. C. Low

References and Notes

1 Manson had demonstrated a very high concentration of embryos (microfilariae) of *Filaria nocturna* in pulmonary histology (obtained at post-mortem) from a West Indian patient in London who suffered from lymphatic filariasis, and who had committed suicide by swallowing prussic acid. (P Manson. On filarial periodicity. *Br med J* 1899; ii: 644–6.)

2 This theme is pursued in a further letter to Manson dated 3 July 1901 (Letter XIII); preliminary results were subsequently published. (*See:* G C Low. The absence of *Anopheles* in Barbadoes, W.I. *Br med J* 1902; i: 200).

3 'Barbados leg' (*See:* J A Simpson, E S C Weiner [eds]. *Oxford English Dictionary* 2nd ed. Oxford: Clarendon Press 1989; 1: 945.)

4 While at Amoy (China) Manson had demonstrated periodicity in *Filaria nocturna* (*Wuchereria bancrofti*) and clearly Low was anxious to confirm this in a different species.

5 The Liverpool School of Tropical Medicine had been officially opened by Lord (Joseph) Lister on 22 April 1899; teaching started the following month. This school had been inaugurated therefore, approximately six months before that in London which was opened to students on 2 October, 1899.

6 This presumably refers to cases of hydrocele and various other abnormalities of the male external genitalia caused by *W. bancrofti*.

7 Individual of mixed ethnic ancestry, i.e. African and Europid. (*See:* J A Simpson, E S C Weiner (eds). *Oxford English Dictionary.* Oxford: Clarendon Press 1989; 10: 68.)

8 Low was to publish these results in 1902 (*Br med J* 1902; i: 1472–3); He was also to refer to these findings in a further paper published several years later. [*See also*: G C Low. Malarial and filarial diseases in Barbadoes, West Indies.

Br Med J 1902; i: 1472–3; G C Low. The unequal distribution of filariasis in the tropics. *Lancet* 1908; i: 279–81.]

9 G C Low. Malarial and filarial diseases in Barbadoes, West Indies. *Br med J* 1902; i: 1472–3.

10 A region of British Guiana (now Guyana) in which a type of raw sugar (the crystals of which have a yellowish-brown colour) was originally produced; the cane was first introduced there in 1848.

11 This description probably refers to an *Echinoderm* – e.g. a starfish or sea-urchin. [*See:* G C Cook, A I Zumla (eds). *Manson's Tropical Diseases* 22nd ed. London: Saunders 2009: 586.]

12 **Sir Frederic Mitchell Hodgson** KCMG (1851–1925) was a highly experienced Colonial Officer. After service on the Gold Coast (now Ghana), he became governor of Barbados (1900–04) and then Governor of British Guiana (now Guyana) (1904–11). [*See also*: Anonymous. Hodgson, Sir Frederic Mitchell. *Who Was Who 1916–1928*. 5th ed. London: A & C Black 1992: 387.]

13 *British Medical Association*. The annual meeting of the BMA in 1901 was held at Cheltenham from 30 July until 2 August. [*See also*: Anonymous. Cheltenham. *J trop Med* 1901; 4: 274–5. This article, while referring to the BMA meeting, concentrates on Cheltenham as a 'health resort'.]

Chapter 6

Mainland South America: two months in British Guiana (Guyana) (July–August 1901)

The next phase of Low's Caribbean venture was a stay of about two months in British Guiana (now Guyana) (*see* Figure 6.1). Here, he continued with his observations on **filariasis**; the question of the vector for *Filaria demarquayi* continued to elude him. He also kept records of the diseases he encountered, especially those amongst the indigenous population. Low's first letter to Manson from Georgetown is dated 13 July 1901.

Letter XIV

Georgetown
B. Guiana
July 13. 01.

Dear Dr. Manson,

I arrived here safely. I am now staying in the hospital with one of the doctors and am getting good work in. I am arranging [?] for Indians, and shall go up [into] the bush and up the coast to get them. I don't think it will be very easy working out the intermediate hosts here unless I could get one in the hospital and strike the right insect which must here be a forest one. *F. Nocturna* abounds; *mosquitos*: *C. taeniatus C. fatigans. Culex* [?] a small black one and any amount of *anopheles*. Larvae of latter very common all through the town in the canals. Georgetown is low lying and the country is in places below sea level, and drained by canals. *Mosquitos* ad libitum and no chance that I can see of [demolishing] them here. The canals are a necessity and they are so numerous you could not [remove] them. It resembles the [Roman] Campagna a little and I should think was as bad as the West Coast of Africa. In the bad districts *mosquito* houses are indicated. I shall study those small filariae carefully but I think

British Guiana

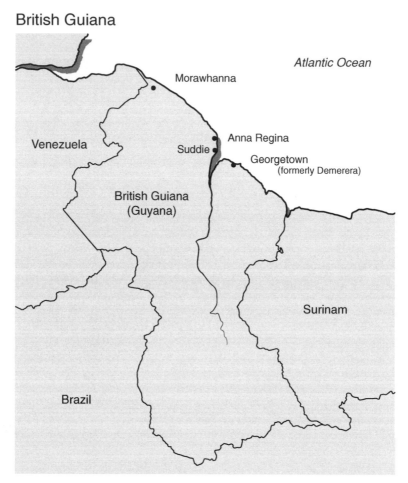

Figure 6.1: Map of British Guiana (now Guyana) showing locations at which Low worked.

the best hope for finding the intermediate host will be St. Vincent [*see* Chapter 7]. The distances are tremendous here and there are no places to stay when you get there. The Indians are nomadic, wandering all over the interior. However I shall try my best and if the sharp tailed turns out be *F. Demarquaii* [sic] I may get some inklings here that will be useful when I get to St. Vincent. I am starting this now as on Tuesday I shall go wandering about the country. The Doctors are all kind and I have the run of the hospital. I have only been here 2 days and already have got much done. I shall keep this open till I leave next week so as to tell you anything of interest that turns up.

I got embryos [microfilarae] in a case of **elephantiasis** to day, a reinfection I suppose. I shall stop now but will add a note before I leave next week. Letters and things still address to Barbados as I go back there from here.

Believe me
Yours sincerely
G. C. Low

No more time just off to the interior.

G. L.

Letter XV

Georgetown
Demerara
July 29.01.

Dear Dr. Manson,

I think this letter will interest you but I am sure you will be disappointed as I was that I have not found that host yet and don't seem much nearer it. I shall just give you a brief account of my doings & first trip to the interior.

Leaving Georgetown one morning at 7 in a steamer I went to a place called Suddie where Dr. Ozzard [*see* Preface] is. I stayed a day and a half there and we had a great time examining specimens. In an Indian in the hosp. there I saw my first B. Guiana sharp tailed filaria and *there is no doubt that it is F.Demarquaii* [sic] [author's italics]. In stained specimens done in exactly the same way as those from the islands one could also see they were the same. Dr Ozzard agreed and so that is one thing settled. The blunt tailed is undoubtedly *F. perstans* tho of course I have not seen the African one alive but still from stained specimens there is no doubt. I left Dr Ozzard, drove 15 miles along the coast, stayed a night with a Dr. at Anna Regina, and next morning embarked in a boat with 5 Indians. We started up a canal and gradually left the cultivated strip of land on the coast and entered the bush; it was very beautiful the trees arching over head formed a tunnel and their stems sank into the dark black water at the sides; beautiful dragon flies and humming birds abounded. The first thing of interest was an attack by *mosquitos*, great big black ones with hairy legs – *Psorophora* or *Sabethes* I think; along with them another species appeared. I got good specimens with ease, the big hairy ones bit through ones clothes with great avidity. We left the strip of bush passed into a very pretty lake, crossed this and rested at the top for a little, and there the crew hauled the boat out of the water over a piece of land and launched it again on the outer side in a creek, really a tributary of the river I was making for. Starting down this the scenery was the same but eventually the water way broadened out, other streams joined, and by afternoon we were in a fairly big river. The bush impenetrable in nature, grass right down to the river and even encroached into it.

Late in the day I arrived at my destination, a police station e.g. a sort of large hut standing on big legs roofed in with a kind of thatch made of big leaves. About 2 miles or so up the river was the Indian settlement I intended to work on. Next morning I visited this, going in a canoe made of the trunk of a tree and which had a tendency for upsetting which I did not care for. I tapped in all 108 Indians and found the enormous percentage of 71 infected, this might have been higher because in several children there were no worms. I then thought the host must be common in such a place & started the Indian boys to catch every insect they could lay [their] hands on at night in the infected huts. The place was specially suitable, the people living in hammocks under what we would call sheds. [?] *mosquitos* at night of most remarkable colours and varieties. The common one was a dark finely built chocolate coloured one with the palps as long as the proboscis in no way resembling an *anopheles* and which I really don't know what to call, probably I should think a new genus all together. It fed quickly but though I dissected over 40 got from infected houses in the vicinity, I did not see a thing in this one. The 2 next in frequency was a big mahogany yellow *culex*. In 2 I found a dead embryo in the semi digested blood in the stomach this shewing [that] they were not efficient. No 3 in frequency a yellow looking *mosquito* with green eyes gave negative results and no 4 a small black *culex* also, but of this [latter] I only got 4 examples. Of course I did not have enough of those latter ones to make absolutely certain, but I am sure if no 1 had been efficient I would have struck embryos in them out of 40 dissections considering over 70 % of the people were infected.

I next turned my attention to fleas dissecting [?] over a dog

P. [*Pulex*] *Irritans* and they were negative. Chiggers[1] abounded and I also went for them. They are as you know terribly small. I mounted several in balsam but have not so far seen anything resembling embryos in them, tho I shall go over them all again carefully. I rather suspect the chigger all the same; could *perstans* have been introduced into Africa with the Chigger?

I put in 5 days of splendid work however, and tho not having found anything very definite still hope for success.

I would have liked to have stayed longer at that place but I had to go back to the coast as the boat a man had kindly lent me was required on a certain day. The subject seems a little different now. *Perstans* was more common a good deal than *Demarquaii* [sic] now; in St. Lucia the focus of greatest prevalence of *D* was Gros Islet a village on sandy ground on the sea coast, chiggers were there undoubtedly. In B. Guiana none of the small filariae are found on the sea coast, only in the interior in the bush amongst the Indians or people who have lived a long time up there.

The *mosquitos* of the interior at the places I was at were all new to me, not in the slightest degree like any in St. Lucia. Of course it does not follow that only one insect spreads it; several may be efficient. I was disappointed really not striking it, but I am just on the eve of departing on trip no 2 to again attack the subject. This time I am going up the Demerara river to another settlement, I shall then see what insects are there and see if any correspond to those already studied. I shall do a week there come back to G.town and then I start on my big expedition to the N.W.

I was very lucky the other day in meeting a Mr. Perkins, one of the boundary commissioners and commissary of the gold mines, a man who knows the interior perfectly. He said he took a great interest in the subject and would be only too glad to collect any material for me, or when I left for the school, if he only knew how to do it. To meet such a man delighted me, and he also asked me to come with him on a 3 weeks journey into the N. West where he is going to inspect a gold mine. At that place I believe many Indians are to be found. I am to shew him how to pin *mosquitos* how to preserve tissues and everything else, and I have not the slightest doubt he will be only too glad to send things home to the school.

We leave G.town on the 8th of August returning on the 26th. On return I shall go back to Barbados stay a little and then go to St. Vincent and go at *Demarquaii* [sic] there. I hope after all this I shall find it. In my intervals in town I have been going at *F. Nocturna* which abounds here. The Drs. have been very kind and have put me up in the hospital where I roam about at night tapping people.

I went to a place one day on the coast called Meldad [sic] said to be the worst place bar one in the colony for *mosquitos*. I sat under a mango tree, and in about 1 minute I was fairly well covered with *anopheles* and 2 species of *culex*, often catching the *anopheles* on one hand [while] they were biting the other like anything. This is the only place I have ever seen them bite like that in the middle of the day. Of course this was under the shade of the aforesaid mango tree.

I have got a lot of specimens for the school. 1st. I send a collection of *mosquitos*, some of them are very rare and quite new. On the inside of the box I have written instructions. The names I want are those marked with little red dots on the discs. I think the best way will be to send them to Theobald [*see* Letter IV]; any thing very rare I think he should keep and not return. If you like, the collection sent and the others I am going to send can be given to the British Museum, or a collection can be started at the school. Whichever way don't let them get destroyed as there will be some exceedingly rare ones and ones not easy to obtain again and I have worked hard to get them. In naming if they refer to the row and description of the insect I shall know which it is. Everything gets so mouldy out here that I am frightened to keep them longer than I can help. Were those *mosquitos* I sent from Barbados with the very long antennae the same as the *Brachiomya* [sic] *magnum* the new species from St. Lucia? I think myself they were.

I address the *mosquitos* to you at Queen Anne Street and in case you are away at your holidays with the additional address of Theobald [*see* above] entomologist British Museum, so that they can be got at once. In addition to those I send

In alcohol. *Mosquitos* (genus ?) from Indian settlement for cutting. I have also kept similar … myself to cut.

2. Screw worms.

3. Ankylostomes.

4. Tissues of granuloma Pudendi.

I hope these all arrive safely, the latter I shall also send to you at Queen Anne Street as I don't suppose there will be anyone at the school in August. I must stop now. I shall not write you next mail as I shall be in the bush but I hope to write the mail after that. I shall do my best and shall collect good material. *Mosquitos* &c.

Dr. Fowler[2] and Dr. Ozzard [*see* Preface] ask me to remember them very kindly to you. They have been uncommonly kind to me out here.

I send some stamps to Miss Manson.

With best regards to Mrs. Manson yourself & family.

Believe me.

Yours sincerely

G. C. Low

Letter XVI

Georgetown

Aug. 28. 01

Dear Dr. Manson,

I have returned safely from the interior and have [had] a very good time amongst the Indians there. In some ways it was not so good as the expedition I told you of on the Pomeroon [formerly Georgetown] River because in the N.W. there is no mission, the natives living here & there in the forest and moving about at pleasure [?]. On account of that I never got a large number at once and could get few insects from the region of their huts. However I got a lot of new tribes, Macusees, Akowolos and Maranio [sic] and found they harboured the same filariae *Demarquaii* [sic] and *Perstans* in large numbers. I think now it [is] a bush *mosquito* that spreads the thing here, and it does not matter what distance one is from the sea as long as the bush is not disturbed.

For example I visited a place on the Demerara river called [?] before going to the N.W. That is a place well up in the interior. Here they had cleared the bush, put up buildings and started a settlement in connection with a gold mine. I examined a great number of half castes, negroes and others who had resided here for periods from 2 to 6 or more years and found some infected with the small filariae. The *mosquitos* prevalent there were *taeniatus, fatigans* and *anopheles albipes* undoubtedly having been introduced from the coast by the steamers that go up there. As against that in the N.W. I examined some Indians near the coast but where the bush had not been disturbed and found they had it. I suspect a metallic blue *mosquito* as having something to do with it as I have found it every where where I have got the filariae. Of course the insect fauna is so enormous that one can not perhaps say definitely and it is impossible to rear those bush *mosquitos* & even to find their larvae. For *Perstans* I think undoubtedly a bush insect spreads it, but for *Demarquaii* [sic] why in St. Lucia should it be found on the coast at Gros Islet and live along with *perstans* in the forests. It will be very interesting now to see the conditions in St. Vincent where I shall go now as soon as possible.

Apart from **filarial diseases** I have got some very useful information with regard to the diseases of the Indians. I never saw any thing resembling **sleeping sickness** and Mr. Perkins [*see* above] with whom I went and who has been all over the interior tells me that he has never seen or heard of it here. He is a trustworthy informant as he has studied your book and knows a lot about those things. **Elephantiasis** is also unknown but one can see how that is because *C. fatigans* the domestic mosquito is not found in the forests. **Malarial fever** is got amongst the Indians and often of a severe type. In that connection it is interesting that in the interior at a place called Criabo [sic] I got an entirely new *anopheles* in large numbers, very small in size. **Ground itch** is very common, this being got on walking in the mud and it [is] evidently due to an acarus which burrows under the skin. I got it myself on a toe, and Perkins got it in his foot. It raises a sort of beeb and I cut those and applied some carbolic which cured it. **Purulent conjunctivitis** and other eye conditions are common [and] spread I am sure by small flies. For example I tapped 15 [?] Indians one day just before coming back to Georgetown; about 8 of those, especially the children, suffered from conjunctivitis with pus in their eyes. Two days after my own eye got sore and I got the same thing with pus coming from my eye, luckily I got to Georgetown and then I had it treated at once with Ag.NO$_3$ [silver nitrate] which has cured it. I noticed at the time dozens of small flies settling on the Indians' eyes and undoubtedly they inoculated me evidently one having settled in my eye after. Another interesting thing is bete [sic] rouge a minute red tick; this bores into ones skin and causes a lot of irritation. I got a plentiful supply of those myself.

For insects of all sorts the places I was in were impossible to beat. I have collected 2 boxes of *mosquitos* many at least to me entirely new and there seems to be no end of them. I am sending these home as it is so damp here and every thing goes bad at once. I marked with little red dots the ones I want the names of specially. If you could get the names for me quoting the box they were in: 1, 2 or 3 I shall know which they were and that will save sending them back. I am sure many have never been got before so it will be best to keep them at home for collections either at the school or the British Museum. As far as that goes the trip has been satisfactory and if I find similar *mosquitos* in St. Vincent in connection with *Demarquaii* [sic] it will give me a clue to go on which should be very useful in determining the host.

It was pretty hard work the journey. I never slept in a bed for 3 weeks. In the bush one sleeps in hammocks, if no house is near under the trees, or if a house exists one ties up one's hammock in the verandah and sleeps there. I am looking forward to [receiving] all my journals and letters on getting back to Barbados on Sunday. I shall work up some material there and go off then to St. Vincent and do that island. I leave here to morrow and arrive there on Saturday. I suppose you have been busy with the *B.M.J.* [author's italics] meeting [*see* Chapter 5]. I am looking forward to see[ing] all that took place there in the journals.

With steamers, boats and walking we covered about 600 miles in the N.W. of B. Guiana.

I am going to give them a paper at the branch of the B.M.A. here to night. I hope you got my paper on **malaria** in Barbados all right. Has the one on **malaria** in St. Lucia appeared yet? I hear Daniels has gone to the West Coast for a trip.[3] I hope they will succeed in the experiments there.

I must stop now but will write you again soon.

Believe me
Yours sincerely
G. C. Low

P.S.
I send the 2 boxes of *mosquitos* per same mail.

G.L.

Low clearly states in this letter that there was no evidence of **trypanosomiasis** (sleeping sickness) in British Guiana (*see also* Chapters 7 and 9). However, *Mansonella perstans* infection was prevalent. It is thus of considerable interest that both Manson and Low felt it worthwhile to investigate the 'negro lethargy' in Uganda with the underlying hypothesis that *M perstans* was the causative organism![4]

References and Notes

1   A 'tropical flea, the female of which burrows and lays eggs beneath the host's skin, causing painful sores. [*Tunga penetrans*]'. (C Soanes, A Stevenson (eds). *Concise Oxford Dictionary* 11th ed. Oxford: Oxford University Press 2006: 246.)

2   **John Francis Scott Fowler** had qualified (MB, CM) from Aberdeen in 1885. He was currently a Government Medical Officer in British Guiana, having previously served as a Surgeon-Captain in the Army. [*See also*: *Medical Directory*. London: J & A Churchill 1902: 1859.]

3   C W Daniels [*see* Letter VIII] had travelled to Sierra Leone, West Africa, to study mosquitoes with the ultimate objective to eliminate malaria – *see* C W Daniels to R Ross. 1 October 1901. In: R Ross. *Mosquito Brigades and how to organise them*. London: George Philip & Son 1902: 92–6.) Daniels had previously studied 'blackwater fever' in east Africa; then, as now, the actual pathogenesis of this entity was unclear, although an association with malaria and quinine was undisputed. [*See also*: G C Cook. Charles Wilberforce Daniels, FRCP (1862–1927): underrated pioneer of tropical medicine. *Acta trop* 2002; 81: 237–50.]

4   G C Cook. Correspondence from Dr George Carmichael Low to Dr Patrick Manson during the first Ugandan sleeping sickness expedition. *J med Biog* 1993; 1: 215–29. [*See also*: G C Cook, A I Zumla (eds). *Manson's Tropical Diseases*. 22nd ed. London: Saunders 2009: 1503–4.]

Chapter 7

Tours of St Vincent, Trinidad and Grenada (September–December 1901)

Following his adventures on the coast and into the interior of British Guiana, Low returned in early September 1901 to Barbados – which continued to be his base. From there he travelled to St Vincent, (and after a further spell in Barbados), Trinidad and Grenada.

Letter XVII

Bay Mansion
Barbados
Sep. 12. 01.

Dear Dr. Manson,
I got back here from Demerara (British Guiana) last week. After arriving I began to feel seedy with aching in my bones and eventually developed malignant **malarial fever** [*P. falciparum* infection]. With energetic treatment by quinine I completely had it under in two days and though tiring easily am all right again. What I disliked most was the enormous perspiration, the weather also at the time being about 90° in the shade. It was interesting in a way. Calculating back I found that 10 days before that I had been at Morawhanna [*see* Figure 6.1] a frightfully unhealthy place in the N.W. of B. Guiana. Most of the people there had suffered from bad fever, and as I slept there in a hammock which I could not properly protect by a *mosquito* net the sequence of events referable to *anopheles* bite is evident. I am glad it had not knocked me up for long as I am going to St. Vincent the day after tomorrow again to pursue *Demarquaii* [sic]. It was interesting to receive your letter with the note, or reprint rather, about **sleeping sickness** and of my paper on Barbados. I got these the day after coming back and I also got the xylol, the fuchsine [sic] and the [?] a day or so ago.

I told you I think I had looked into the **sleeping sickness** question in B. Guiana whilst amongst the Indians. I could not hear [of] or see any cases of the disease there and no one, bushmen and others, had heard of it, I don't think it probably can exist there at all although as I told you there is plenty [of] *filaria perstans*.[1]

Since coming back here I have not had time to do much owing to the fever but I again inspected many parts of the island, namely the Worthing swamps [at the south-west of the island] and other pools of water. The conditions were just the same as before not the trace of an *anopheles* and this time hardly any *culex*. A point bearing on the absence of **malaria** in Barbados I picked up in B. Guiana, namely that the Barbadian negro when there suffers very severely from the Demerara fevers, more so than the indigenous negro of those parts, this I suppose means he is [in] the same position as the white man who comes from home e.g. has not had the means of attaining any immunity.[2] I am to take a good supply of the swamp water over to St. Vincent with me and shall try if *anopheles* larvae can live in it, as you suggested.

I am looking forward with special interest to the localisation of *Demarquaii* [sic] in that island and the insects to be found there. I examined 12 jiggers [chiggers] which I got and mounted in the Pomeroon river [*see* Chapter 6] in Demerara the other day. Those came from infected cases but I could not see anything in them at all. I don't think now the jiggers is the host. I would like very much if Theobald [*see* Letter IV] could send me the names of some of the *mosquitos* I mailed with red dots from B. Guiana. I think a metallic blue one [*see* Chapter 6] is high suspicious and if I find the same in St. Vincent it will strengthen this.

I read Theobald's paper on the classification of *mosquitos*, founded on the scales &c and I have been going into that and find it interesting and very instructive. I am sure many of the insects I sent from B. Guiana are quite new all together, and I hope all the collections got safely home. The little *anopheles* from Corcato [?] is new and the dark *mosquito* from the Pomeroon with the palps as long as the proboscis though having the wing scales [of] an *anopheles* is I think a new genus all together. If he could send me names as soon as possible it would help me with my work. I shall start a new collection in St. Vincent to send home as soon as possible and those I should also like named and classified as in all probability one or other must be hosts. I hope I shall find the thing now all right and settle the matter.

I must stop now as I have nothing more to say.

Address letters still to Bay Mansion, Barbados as they forward to me wherever I am.

Believe me,

Ever Yours Sincerely

G. C. Low

Letter XVIII

St. Vincent WI.

Sep. 25. 01.

Dear Dr. Manson,

As things were not very busy after my fever I started a paper on *F. Demarquaii* [sic] in Barbados, and have now finished it here.[3] I have put in all I have been able to find out about the subject and as you will see from it I think the sharp tailed B. Guiana filaria is the same, and have described it as so and gone into the prevalence & host question. If you think it worth it, you might send it to the *B.M.J.* [author's italics] or, if not, to the tropical journal as I have not written anything for them yet. You will read it and see what you think.

In addition to this I have sent you a note for the correspondence columns of the *B.M. Journal* [author's italics] on the fact of *anopheles* larvae in St. Vincent living & growing in the swamp water of Barbados which I took over. I think this is interesting & worth publishing.[4]

I got over here last week [*see* Figure 7.1] and after being kept in the house for two day[s] owing to a storm with tremendous rain eventually got started. Dr. Newsam shewed me the list you sent to him in [18]94 and on consulting it I found Jane Pemberton was still living & resided in a village 3 miles from Kingstown. I started for there at once and found the place to be a village on swampy sandy ground with scrubby bush around & about & very little cultivation, not unlike Gros Islet in St. Lucia in someways, though with hills close behind. Jane Pemberton has still got the embryos [microfilariae of *W bancrofti*] in abundance & I sent a box to Daniels [*see* Letter VIII] for the school, full of slides. I tapped 28 people besides & found 8 infected some with many so the village is an infected area all right. Search for insects revealed the common … *anopheles* larvae,

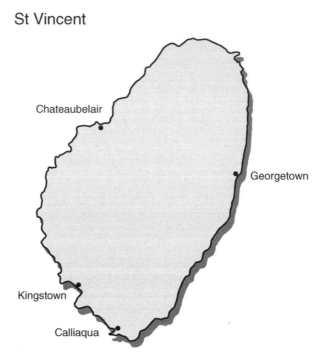

St Vincent

Chateaubelair

Georgetown

Kingstown

Calliaqua

Figure 7.1: Map of St Vincent, showing locations at which Low worked.

and insects collected were all common, with the exception of a new *culex* resembling *taeniatus*. Several of this [?] from Mrs Pemberton's bed room gave neg. results.

I spent a whole afternoon there trekking about and asked the people about insects. Sandflies are common but so far I could not get any details of different *mosquitos*. The host is more difficult than I expected and whether or not I shall ever find it I do not know. I must just go on dissecting insects of all sorts in detail and hope to strike it that way. Another difficulty is the rearing of sand flies & insects like that, or even the rarer genera of *mosquitos* from larvae, and even the keeping of such insects alive for more than a day or so. Still if one could find an insect several times infected from an infected house one would get a very definite clue & this I hope to do. I have got a staff of boys busily catching every *mosquito* they can see and also all sorts of larvae, and to morrow I go for the day there and again to inspect.

There is no place to stay in unfortunately, but I shall see the administrator and suggest that I stay for a night or so in the policeman's quarters. I have got through a lot of the districts already & have been going well for the short time I have been here. I went down the leeward coast yesterday, stayed a night and tapped 2 villages.

The heat is the trying part of the business as it is about its worst now and it is simply like being in a vapour bath all day. As it is the hurricane season one never knows what is going to happen. There was a tremendous storm lasting the whole day last week but luckily unaccompanied by wind. The island is a pretty one like St. Lucia. Dr. Newsam [*see* Chapter 4] is very kind in doing what he can to help me, and the Administrator also has promised every help.

On Saturday I do the windward side of the island to see if the worm is got there and … then I shall have been pretty well over the whole island. You will see in the paper I send, the details about *Demarquaii* [sic]; I hope it arrives safely. You will see what you think of it when you read it. I have not seen the malarial paper on St. Lucia yet[5] but I suppose they are pressed for room at present.

With best regards
Believe me
Yours Sincerely
G. C. Low

Letter XIX

Kingstown
St. Vincent
Oct. 7. 01.

My dear Dr. Manson,
I got your last letter all right, sent on from Barbados, and was glad to get all your news and to hear of your shooting expedition. With the exception of 2 flamingoes and an ibis which I shot in B. Guiana I have done nothing in that line.

I think I told you in my last letter that I was beginning to doubt about finding the intermediate host of *F. Demarquaii* [sic] and my work here I am sorry to say has strengthened that view. In the paper I sent you home last mail you would see a description of Calliaqua the place where the filaria is specially found. Well, I made a most exhaustive and thorough examination of this village spending several whole days & evenings in it and searched every inch of water about the place for larvae. There were plenty [of] *anopheles* about and **malarial fever**, so I thought I would just rear some of those again and get them to bite infected people. I did *A. Albipes* and *argyritarsis* but failed to find the faintest trace of filariae in them after the blood had been digested from the stomach. This confirmed the results of St. Lucia. Of other mosquitos there, *C. fatigans* & *taeniatus* were common and 2 genera of Crab hole mosquitos. *Brachiosoma* & *Dermeeritesv* [sic] those latter 2 frequent houses all right but though examining a large number I never found blood in them and have never been [able to] get them to bite in captivity. I don't think they bite at all. I heard of a blue *mosquito* but it is not got near this village and most of the people have never been in the district in which it is found.

The annoying [thing] is the disease is quite common in Calliaqua and one would suppose the intermediate host must also be common. Those are the *mosquitos* of the place and of other insects I could find nothing definite, nor hear of the people being specially bitten by any.

There are sandflies but at this season of the year, very few. Of *Muscidae* there are no biting examples, and of *Tabanidae* ditto. Bugs might have something to do with it then their distribution is general everywhere, not being specially limited to that place. As I say I found no other species of *mosquito* there but might of course have missed one, but in that case it must be very rare and then that would not likely be the host of the filaria when it is so prevalent there. Could the worm escape any other way do you think? I examined urine in cases with negative results. One point about it is that old people especially the old women have it most. The fact of those latter always sitting about house is suggestive. From the point of its extremely localised distribution I should say it must be a rare or a generally closely distributed insect. What do you think?

I have been over the whole island and have finished it now. Ordinary **filarial disease** is as in the other hilly islands about 6%. **Malaria** is not common, only one or two swampy parts having it, and all things considered the island is, after Barbados, one of the healthiest I have been in.

As I cannot get much work here I am going back to Barbados at the end of the week as I have some materials I want to cut sections of, and I also want to try and get post mortem examinations of *filaria nocturna* cases. I also hope after the Governor gets the letter from the Colonial Office at home, to see about trying to destroy *culex* in that place. I hope to stay a fortnight there and then I shall go to Trinidad and work it out. Ordinary **filarial disease** is prevalent there and I expect I shall find *Demarquaii* [sic] if not *perstans* also, as I believe the bush there is very similar to B. Guiana. I shall try and have a look at Grenada coming from there. *F. Demarquaii* [sic] is almost certain to be found there, as the island resembles St. Vincent.

A lot of the villages here that do not have *Demarquaii* [sic] resemble Calliaqua closely, with the exception that they are not swampy and do not have **malarial fever**, but then conversely to that is the case of Anse-la-raye in St. Lucia [*see* Chapter 4] which is swampy, full of **malaria** and yet does not have *Demarquaii* [sic].[6] Can you suggest any further procedure in the quest for it? You can write and let me know, and also what you think I should now do.

I had an experience the other day coming from Georgetown on the windward side back to Kingstown. I got caught in a storm and got almost drowned in the rain. It was so bad it soaked all my baggage and [my] filaria register book was like pulp when I got home, and my slide box dissolved into bits. I managed to dry my book carefully and it is not much the worse now and I got a new box made here in wood instead of in cardboard. This island is very poor after the hurricane, and they do not have more than 20 or 30 patients in hospital [*see* Figure 7.2] many of those being old chronic ulcers, a subject [on] which a good lot of work could be done.

Yaws exist[s] but it is not notified and they have no hospital for it. I read a paper by a man in Fiji on **yaws** the other day in a blue book on Colonial Medical reports. In many points it seems to differ from the **yaws** here. Our weather has been terribly hot lately and there are bad storms coming every now and then. I hope I don't get caught in the centre or hurricane part of one. The last bad hurricane here killed over 200 people, knocked down thousands of houses and cleared the island pretty well of trees. The hurricane season will be over by the end of the month and then the weather becomes settled again.

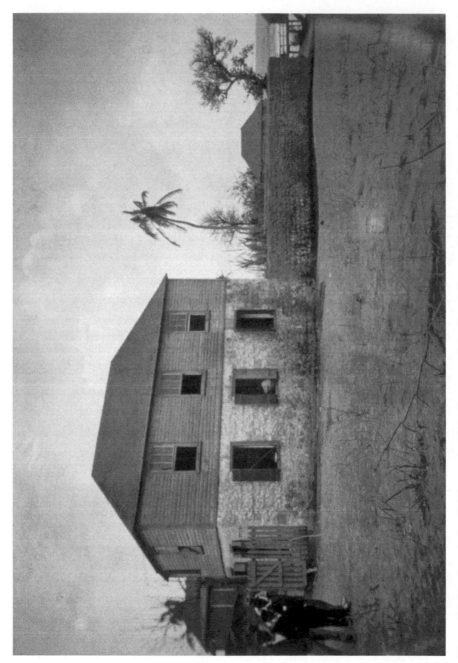

Figure 7.2: The hospital at St Vincent in 1902. Courtesy of the Royal Geographical Society (reproduced with permission).

I was interested to read of your son's relapse of his **malarial fever** [a *P vivax* infection] when in Aberdeen and also of Warrens relapses.[7] It shews how persistent the parasite is and also that it must have a latent life somewhere in the spleen or internal organs.[8] Those cases not having been subject to reinfection shew this very well. I hope you will have a good session this autumn and plenty [of] good cases. If I can hear of anyone with *Demarquaii* [sic] embryos likely to go home I shall see that he goes to you. There was a little white boy in St. Lucia with them who I expect will go home to school in a year or so.

I must stop now as my stock of news is exhausted.

I send your daughter some stamps.

With best regards to Mrs. Manson Yourself and family.

Believe me,

Yours Sincerely

G. C. Low

Letter XX

Bay Mansion

Barbados

Oct. 11. 01.

Dear Dr. Manson,

I got back … here [Barbados] this morning. I went into the village of Calliaqua though after my letter to you went from St. Vincent but could find nothing definite. At a place Chateaubelair I found no *Demarquaii* [sic] cases but I got a blue *mosquito* there, I think the *Haemagogus* of Milistonia, it resembles one I saw in B. Guiana. I shall send a box of St. Vincent specimens next mail.

I heard from Dr. Galgey [*see* Letter I] the other day that he had got some parents of *Demarquaii* [sic] in St. Lucia and I advised him to mount them in glycerine jelly and send them to you. This ought to clear the matter up.

I hope you got my paper all right. I have just read Dutton's paper on the escape of the filaria from the proboscis.[9] I think his explanation is good & better than Grassi's. I must stop as the mail is just going.

The Governor [Sir Frederic Hodgson – *see* Letter XIII] should soon

[hear] from the colonial office now and then I hope he will start to rid this place of *mosquitos*. I have not seen him lately.

Ever Yours Sincerely

G. C. Low

Letter XXI

Bay Mansion.

Barbados.

Oct. 25. 01.

My dear Dr. Manson,

Just a line to let you know how things go on here. I have been working in Barbados for the last fortnight since returning from St. Vincent. I have been cutting sections and going into detailed studies of **filarial cases**, the latter being very interesting.

I have had a good run lately and again got a case with a first attack of filarial lymphangitis. Many examinations of his blood shew no embryos and I suppose the parents have died, and in so dying have set up inflammation. I should think provided no reinfection takes place that the first should also be his last attack, ie if the death of the parents is correct.

Those cases are very interesting and it would be very nice if one could only get post mortem examinations to help me, but unfortunately they will not die. At present I have 2 cases of **elephantiasis** neither of which have ever had lymphangitis or as they call it here 'fever and ague'. They just began slowly to form and one is quite early, and interesting to say I found 2 embryos in her blood out of 6 slides examined. Of course they may come from parents situated at some other part of her body. I think myself they get reinfected time after time as most will not sleep under *mosquito* nets. I saw the Governor [Hodgson] the other day and he said he wanted to do something to try and diminish it. He thought a series of pamphlets to the schools and other places would be a good thing. It will require persistent training to get the people to understand the thing.

I am going to Trinidad on Monday as I wish to finish off that island & Grenada & I want to see how they are situated as regards **filariasis** and specially to note if *Demarquaii* [sic] exists there, and to have another try at the host. After I do them I shall return here, as

I get very good facilities for the study of cases at the hospital and I find this is the best place to make my headquarters. I expect to be away for a month or 6 weeks and on returning will see what is to be done as regards the destruction of *mosquitos* and the best means of getting the people interested. I have seen most of the pathological stages of *nocturna* here and want to get notes, temperatures, and clinical facts about them & hope also for post mortems in some cases I have my eye on.

There is a very interesting disease here which they call **Psilosis pigmentosa**.[10] I think it is the same as the Italian **pellagra**. It is got in the poor natives but the alimentary symptoms are very like your description of the East Indian psilosis which I have gone carefully through. Briefly this disease then is got in the poor. They get an erythema on the dorsum of the hands and this becomes pigmented but before this is papular. This is like **pellagra** disease in Italy. After that wasting begins. The tongue is red and shews ulceration round the edges, and they get chronic diarrhoea. Pigmentary patches may now appear on the face & on the extensor surface of the knees. They go down hill fairly rapidly & towards the end most go mad and die insane. Taken all over it resembles very closely the **pellagra** I saw in Italy, and some Italian surgeons from a Man of War at once diagnosed it as that.

I shall get tissues and post mortems on coming back from Trinidad & send you material to the school, as well as working at it here. Most of my last sections were poor as my celloidin had absorbed water from the air and had gone bad. I was taking photos of **elephantiasis** cases yesterday, but the plates owing to the same moisture in the air were bad & the prints are poor. I shall take more however.

I hope to get some good work in Trinidad & Grenada. I send you a box of *mosquitos* I collected in St. Vincent this mail. I have had similar specimens from St. Lucia and there is nothing new with the exception of the metallic blue one which is the *Haemagogus* [of] Milistonia [*see* Letter XX] I believe. Theobald [*see* Letter IV] however will know. I shall write him a note telling him about it.

I must stop now as it is near mail time.

With best regards to Mrs. Manson and your family.

Believe me

Yours Sincerely

G. C. Low

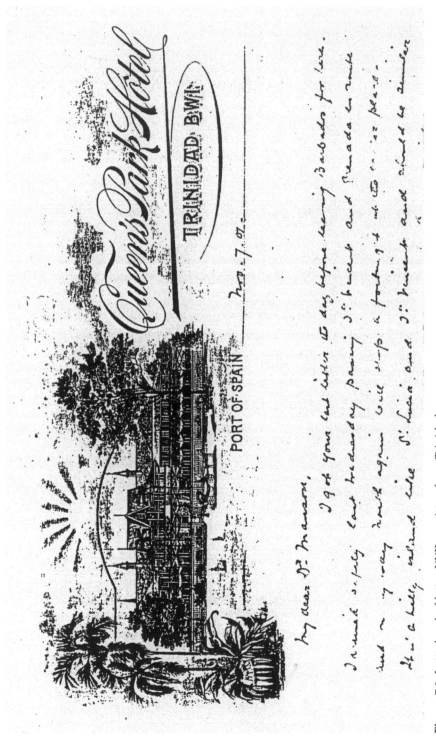

Figure 7.3: Letterhead of letter XXII – written from Trinidad.

Letter XXII

Queen's Park Hotel [*see* Figure 7.3]
Trinidad B.W.I.
Port of Spain
Nov. 7. 01.

My dear Dr. Manson,

I got your last letter the day before leaving Barbados for here. I arrived safely last Wednesday passing St. Vincent and Grenada en route and on my way north again will stop a fortnight at the latter place. It is a hilly island like St. Lucia and St. Vincent and should be similar as regards **Filarial diseases** I think. This place is a very fine one and there is as you see from the above picture a decent hotel which one does not find in the small islands, the accommodation there being miserable in the extreme. I found all the people glad to see me. I dined at Government House one night, and the Governor was interested and promised me every facility. The acting Surgeon General a Dr. De-Wolf also made things easy, so I got started to work the second day after arrival in their laboratory at the hospital.

The hospital is large, and they have a nice little laboratory with facilities for bacteriological and other work, a position much in advance of the other islands with the exception of British Guiana. What delighted me most was to find that the Doctors at the hospital go in for research work and laboratory work to a certain extent, and one man at St. Vincent has been doing some work at **filarial diseases**. I took most interest in him and had a look at some specimens of his bearing on filaria. He told me that after seeing my St. Lucia paper[11] he began & worked at inspecting *mosquitos* and found the same results. But what will interest you most is the following. Some time ago he got a case of *Filaria Demarquaii* [sic] and he tried the various insects he could get on it. I daresay you remember me telling you that in one instance I got a sausage stage in the muscle of a *taeniatus* fed on a *Demarquaii* [sic] case but never finding it again considered it must have been a contamination with *nocturna*. Well he told me that when he started he got in his first *taeniatus* a sausage stage and the person only had *Demarquaii* [sic]. Going at this he dissected 30 more examples but never found a later development, and in only two did he ever see … the sausage stage. He infected 3 *taeniatus* on the *Demarquaii* [sic] case the other day and in one again got a sausage stage just like I noticed in St. Lucia. This I think is very interesting. Of course the results show *taeniatus* is inefficient but I think from the fact of the filaria in rare instances being found in the muscle of that insect and shewing some developments, that it points that it develops in the muscle of its non efficient host whatever insect that may be and probably not in the people it bites. This is a clue therefore and is interesting. His other results also corroborate mine, he also having excluded *fatigans* and another *mosquito* and he further fed bugs on the case excluding them, an insect I had not done.

In addition to this [Doctor] Vincent has done analysis of the prevalence of **filarial disease** here, and though I am doing it all over again I dont expect to find much difference from his figures. I think it will come out at about 10%, the lowness being due to the fact that the town is well drained & has very few water tubs or old wells about it.

Outside of the town … the country is very swampy and plenty [of] **malaria** exists. I am happy to say that here again the men are working, and one I believe has a good collection of the *mosquitos*. The case of *Demarquaii* [sic] has never been out of the island & comes from a village on the North Coast somewhere but I have not had time to go there yet. I have done one village near town & did not find it but once I finish the hospital bloods I shall start on the country districts. I shall write you next mail telling you results.

Believe me
Yours sincerely
G. C. Low

Letter XXIII

Port of Spain
Trinidad
Nov. 16th 01.

My dear Dr. Manson,
I was very glad to get your letter of last mail, sent onto me here from Barbados. I have practically finished Trinidad now, and find it resembles the other smaller and hilly islands more than the mainland [British Guiana]. The hilly portion in the north and the leeward coast of the island which is flat extends right down the island to the

south. I have examined 400 people's blood by night and about 70 day bloods from villages and find that *perstans* is absent, *nocturna* present in 18% of the people ie. less than Barbados, while *Demarquaii* [sic] is also absent in the flat part of the island i.e. resembling the flat and coastal part of Demerara. The only case of indigenous *Demarquaii* [similar] to one [in] St. Vincent has in the [?] and he comes from a village called [?] right in the north at the base of [?]; this place [I have] not been able to get to as the steamers only go once a week and are away 4 days and they may only stop at Matelot [*see* Figure 7.4] half an hour depending on the amount of cargo they are to ship. This however does not matter as the description of the place is similar to the places in the other hilly islands. I have been trying to get more cases in the hospital here from Matelot but I have not yet succeeded in doing so. Large numbers of the 400 cases [come] from all over the island and none from any of these places have it. I got it in another case but he had lived in Dominica.

Trinidad

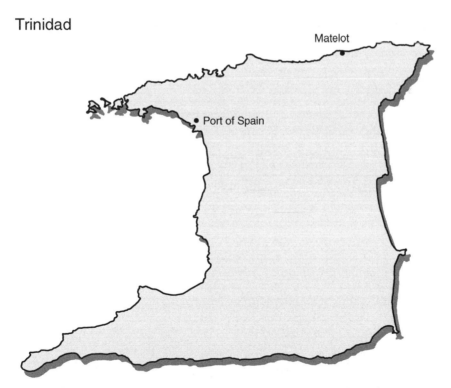

Figure 7.4: Map of Trinidad, showing Matelot – where Low carried out further researches.

Conclusions therefore *Nocturna* common. *Demarquaii* [sic] rare only so far in Matelot on the sea coast at the base of the hills. *Perstans* absent. *Mosquitos* similar to hilly islands, and in the flat swampy ground on the leeward coast, some the same as in Demerara [*see* Chapter 6]. The only important point then here is the fact I told you off [sic] in last letter of the appearance of a rare slightly developed form in the muscles of *Taeniatus* in rare instances. This showing that in the proper host it probably develops here. **Malaria** is very common here. 1 mile from the town there is an enormous swamp full of *anopheles*. The town is practically free of it, is well drained and there are no collections of water in it suitable for *anopheles* breeding.

I go to Grenada on Thursday. I saw [it] in coming here. It is a hilly island and I am sure from the look of it *Demarquaii* [sic] will be present. I hope therefore to get another clue. I shall stay a fortnight there and then back to Barbados. After 2 days waiting there for the home mail, I shall go to St. Kitts and polish it off.

It is rather a bother going to it as it is a long journey and from what I can hear is healthy, and I just wanted to start the extirpation of *mosquitos* in Barbados, but I shall postpone that till I get back which should be about the 20th of December. I agree with you that they should pay my expenses for going all that distance to inspect the place but of course I shall not mention that to them. I saw a man here one day who knew the island and it seems there is a swamp near the town and I expect their '**yellow fever** cases', malignant **malaria** I expect, come from there. I shall see if it is practicable to fill up this swamp and shall condemn those privies mentioned in the letter you sent me. The latter will be useful also in getting an idea of what to expect.

I am quite keen on the killing off [sic] the Barbados *mosquitos*. By now you will have got the correspondence bet. myself and the government of that place on the subject. Those pamphlets are to be distributed on the island and that will be good for a start. The Governor [Hodgson] is keen about it also and when I get back from St. Kitts I shall see him and suggest some more plans. I think a series of lectures to the Sanitary Inspectors, would be a good thing and then a systematic visit of the town say in company with the head of that department. I can then point out the breeding places shewing them what is required to be done, and after that if necessary they can pass a law to have old wells filled up and water tubs condemned. I don't [think] the expense ought to be much. The main difficulty may be their legislative council which is composed of Barbadians who cannot see the good of such measures but the Governor should be able to overcome that. I shall see also what the probable expense will be and then the Colonial Office at home if there are difficulties can see to that. If they act on the simple suggestions, a lot of good I am sure can be done. I am sorry I cant start sooner but I must do Grenada & St. Kitts first and get them out of the way.

I think the Liverpool people are trumpeting a little too loud just at present, they might at least wait a little till they see how things turn out on the West Coast.[12] Of course if they have plenty [of] money and the houses lend themselves to effective drainage and sanitation much good will be done, but that will not deal with forests and large swamps in the country where Europeans have to live and which are full of *anopheles*. I shall do my best [to] keep the name of the London School up to the mark out here.

I was interested in the expedition to Christmas Island and I hope your son[13] and Durham[14] will do well at it. I was sorry I missed seeing Durham when he passed Barbados after coming from Para.

I hope my papers will appear soon in the *B.M. Journal* [author's italics] but I suppose they have lots to put in. I think probably the differences bet. the Demerara parental forms and the ones Galgey [*see* Letter I] sent are probably due to difference[s] of mounting. At least if they are so like as you say and the embryos are also identical it is difficult to see how they can be different. The only point I can see any difference in is the places they are found in, as certainly the bush of Demerara is not like the places I have found them in the small islands, but still the same insect probably is found in both these places.

I forgot when on Trinidad to say I found *F. nocturna* in the common *anopheles*. They develop well in them but I have never been able to keep them a long enough time alive to get them in the proboscis. The same Doctor Vincent [*see* above] I told you off [sic] kept them 11 days alive & then the embryos were almost mature. From what we know of the *anopheles* James[15] in India worked with, it is clear however that they are efficient hosts though undoubtedly the commonest disseminator of the disease out here is *C. fatigans*.

I have met some very nice people in Trinidad, a Mr Justice

Routledge[16] said he came from Aberdeen and said I think he knew you. Chief Justice Baynes also said he had seen you when home. Taken all over Port of Spain their [major] town is healthy for the tropics, and people who do not have to go in the country are remarkably free from fevers.

I saw a lot of **yaws** the other day. I saw a short note on **forest yaws**, the thing I sent you a specimen of from St. Lucia, in the Tropical journal one day, I think by a Dutchman. It is the same disease as the man I saw in St. Lucia; funnily I never saw it in Demerara [*see* Chapter 6] or in people who had lived in the forests there. The man in St. Lucia had got his in the forests of Cayenne [French Guiana]. **Leprosy** is common here and they have a large asylum which I saw the other day.

It is frightfully hot in Trinidad as the town is shut in by hills to the north. It is funny to think of you all at home probably shivering in snowstorms and frost, while sitting here in this moist heat.

I must stop now as I have exhausted my stock of news.

I shall let you hear from Grenada how I fare there.

With best regards to Mrs. Manson and your family and yourself.

Believe me

Yours sincerely

G. C. Low

P.S. I send you[r] daughter a few stamps.

Letter XXIV

Grenada [*see* Figure 7.5]

Dec. 7. 01.

Dear Dr. Manson,

I have not much time left for this mail but as it is the Christmas one I do not want to let it pass without writing to you. I have done a tremendous 14 days work having finished Grenada in that time.

I arrived on a Friday morning and started at once by tapping 100 people that night. Next night I did 50 and the day after started to go round all the villages in the island. I went to a place called Gouyave first and on arrival drove with the Dr. to Victoria another village 5 miles off, tapped 25 people there, then went back to Gouyave and

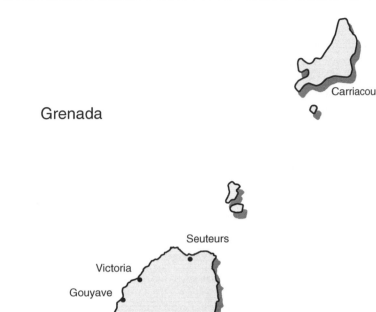

Figure 7.5: Map of Grenada and Carriacou showing locations at which Low worked.

stayed the night tapping the people of that place in the evening. Next day I left in the steamer and went on to the next place, Seuteurs, right at the north of the island. I rode 5 miles into the country and stayed the night with the Dr. then went back to the village next day, examined swamps and bloods and met the steamer at 3 in the afternoon. On board were the Colonial Secretary, the Col. Surgeon and 4 other Government officials and I went in company with them to inspect Carriacou, one of the Grenadine islands half way bet. St. Vincent and Grenada, a place notorious for its *anopheles*. We got off it at 8 P.M., had dinner and then I went on shore to examine bloods. I got those and also plenty [of] *anopheles* and then back on board and slept the night.

Next day we all went on shore to inspect the hospital which is unhealthy, people getting fever after being in it for 10 days or so. The cause was simple, 2 large swamps accounting for this. I advised them to change the site & make it *mosquito* proof with wire netting. After this we rode and looked at a proposed new site a mile and a half off. There were no swamps there, and the ground was sandy and the people live there in safety. It was splendid proof again of the *mosquito* as the spreading agent, and every day of ones life out here one sees the same thing exemplified. In the afternoon I rode around and over the island and then we left at night getting back to St. George's the [major] town of Grenada at 11 at night. I inspected swamps near that town next day and then the next day rested and examined my bloods. The following day I started to cross the island to do the last village. I rode with the inspector of works to the ridge of the island 200 feet high and spent the night on what is called the Grand Etang at a rest house there. Next morning we started early and went down a beautiful valley to the village called Grenville. I had breakfast with the Doctor but then went to inspect the place. I tapped 30 people, found plenty [of] *Anopheles* in the marshes, then started for home in the afternoon riding right over the island back to St. Georges. I dined with the medical men that evening.

Worked next day examining bloods and gave a lecture at night. I gave them **malaria** & **filariasis** and had a very good audience, the Col. Secretary who is acting for the Governor being in the Chair. I dealt with … prevention fully and I think they appreciated it. To day I finish up and leave to morrow for Barbados en route for St. Kitts, do that place then back to Barbados to work at the extermination of *mosquitos*.

I think I have put in a very fair 2 weeks work here and my results are exceedingly interesting shewing that **filariasis** is extremely rare and that *F. Demarquaii* [sic] does not exist [or] at least I have not found it though I have done all the villages and towns.

Results: 175 night examinations no filaria. 276 night or day, no *Demarquaii* [sic]. *Filaria nocturna* does and can exist as *C. fatigans* is present.

I got one case of varicose glands and **elephantiasis** combined yesterday that had never been out of the island to prove that. I also found embryos in a Barbadian who had just come. The % of infection for the island is under 1% a most interesting fact. I don't think though some of the villages looked suitable [for] *Demarquaii* [sic] [to be] present. I examined sufficient people in all these places to practically exclude it with certainty, and this makes it more interesting than ever. I did not find it in Carriacou, the Grenadine[s] and only one case of *nocturna* there, a St. Kitts native.

This coincides with the clinical experience of the Doctors of both islands who rarely see cases of **Filarial disease** and those they do see are generally **elephantiasis** cases from Barbados.

I heard yesterday that **yellow fever**[17] had broken out in St. Lucia, 6 cases [including] 2 deaths I think this is probably true **yellow fever** and not **malaria** as Gray [*see* Letter I] I am sure would examine the blood for parasites. If it spreads I might go there and see it and do something at its prevention by getting them to destroy *C. fasciatus* [*Aëdes aegypti*] which the Americans have found to spread it.[18] The worst is I might get kept there for a long time because no other island would admit me; they have already quarantined St. Lucia.

I hope to get on [with] the examination of the *mosquitos* when I can get back to Barbados.

I hope you are keeping well and that things are going on well at home. I met a Dr. Statham[19] here who had [undertaken] the course. I must stop now as it is just time to post for the mail.

I send Miss some Grenada stamps and also Mrs. Manson a Christmas P.C which I hope arrives.

With best wishes for a merry Xmas and a happy New Year to all of you at Queen Anne Street.

Believe me.
Yours sincerely
G. C. Low

References and Notes

1 Manson, who was at that time virtually obsessed with various forms of filariasis, believing that numerous *tropical* diseases were caused by them, considered that *Filaria perstans* was the probable *cause* of 'negro lethargy' (East African trypanosomiasis) which was sweeping the northern shore of Lake Victoria Nyanza. [*See*: G C Cook. Correspondence from Dr George Carmichael Low to Dr Patrick Manson during the first Ugandan sleeping sickness expedition. *J med Biog* 1993; 1: 215–29.]
2 This is a further reference to Low's interest in relative 'immunity' to the human malarias.

3 G C Low. Notes on Filaria demarquaii. *Br med J* 1902; i: 196–7.

4 The author has found no evidence that this paper was ever published. [*See also*: Chapter 10.]

5 St G Gray, G C Low. Malarial fever in St Lucia. *Br med J* 1902; i: 193–4.

6 G C Low. The unequal distribution of filariasis in the tropics. *Lancet* 1908; i: 279–81. G C Low. The unequal distribution of filariasis in the tropics. *Trans Soc trop Med Hyg* 1908; 1: 84–96. [*See also*: *Op cit*. See Note 3 above.]

7 This refers to a *P. vivax* infection which had been induced (during July–September 1900) in P T ('Burnie') Manson (son of Sir Patrick) (*see* below) and Warren (the laboratory technician at the LSTM) by infected mosquitoes sent from Italy; Manson's first 'relapse' occurred whilst he was in Aberdeen during the summer of 1901 and the second whilst he was shooting in September 1901. Warren's 'relapse' occurred 9 months after the original infection. The infections ultimately responded to quinine chemotherapy.

8 It was not until 1948, when H E Shortt and his colleagues identified the hypnozoite stage of *P vivax* in the human liver that this latent phase in the life-cycle of the parasite was clearly delineated. [*See also*: H E Shortt, P C C Garnham, G Covell, P G Shute. The pre-erythrocytic stage of human malaria, *Plasmodium vivax*. *Br med J* 1948; i: 547.]

9 The author is unable to locate a reference to this work.

10 This probably refers to the desquamating rash on exposed parts seen in pellagra. Psilosis: 'to strip bare, make bald (Greek)'. [*See*: J A Simpson, E S C Weiner (eds). *The Oxford English Dictionary* 2nd ed. Oxford: Clarendon Press 1989; 12: 754.]

11 *Op cit*. See Note 3 above.

12 This presumably refers to malaria control. Following Ross's pioneering work in India which had unravelled the rôle of the mosquito in the *Proteosoma* life-cycle, this became the dominant theme of the Liverpool School of Tropical Medicine. [*See also*: Chapter 8.]

13 **Patrick Thurburn Manson** (1878–1902) was the eldest son of (Sir) Patrick Manson. He left England for Christmas Island in January 1902. Whilst investigating beri-beri, he was tragically killed on 8 March 1902 in a shooting accident; some consider this to have been suicide. Manson (senior), who had organised the expedition, apparently never referred publicly to this event, and it is of interest that he does not mention it in any of this correspondence; the episode is *not* mentioned in any of Low's letters.

14 **Herbert Edward Durham** (1870–1945) later became a distinguished bacteriologist and microbiologist. Based at the Pathological Laboratory, Cambridge, he had studied at Cambridge, Vienna, and Guy's Hospital, qualifiying MB (Camb), BS in 1892; two years later, he had obtained the FRCS (England). Durham had published extensively. [*See also*: *Medical Directory*. London: J & A Churchill 1902: 762.]

15 **Sydney Price James** FRS (1872–1946), working at Travancore, India, had confirmed Low's work which clearly demonstrated microfilariae in the proboscis sheath of *Culex* mosquitoes, in 1900. This confirmed the route of

mosquito-man transmission of lymphatic filariasis, previously considered to be from mosquito-contaminated drinking-water. [*See also*: Anonymous. James, Lt-Col. Sydney Price. *Who Was Who 1941–1950*. 5th ed. London: A & C Black 1980: 596–7.]

16 **Robert Routledge** (??–1907) was educated at Aberdeen University and called to the Bar in 1879. From 1901–06 he was Puisne Judge for Trinidad. [*See also*: Anonymous. Routledge, Robert M. *Who Was Who 1897–1915*. 5th ed. London: A & C Black 1966: 614.]

17 Yellow fever was at that time endemic in the central Americas, having probably been introduced by West African slaves who were imported to run the sugar industry. The West Indies had often been referred to as the 'British Sugar Islands'. [*See also*: R S Dunn. *Sugar and slaves: the rise of the planter class in the English West Indies 1624–1713*. Chapel Hill: University of North Carolina Press 1972: 359.]

18 The American Yellow Fever Commission expedition led by Walter Reed (1851–1902) had recently clinched transmission of the infection by the *Aëdes aegypti* (*C. fasciatus*) mosquito. The report of the Commission was first published at the Annual Congress of the American Public Health Association held at Indianapolis on 22–26 October 1900, but the results only became widely known in early 1901. [*See also*: G Williams. *The Plague Killers*. New York: Charles Scribner's Sons 1969: 345.]

19 No reference can be found to Dr Statham in the *Medical Directory*. London: J & A Churchill, for the relevant period.

Chapter 8

Yellow fever at St Lucia (December 1901–January 1902)

At this point in his expedition, Low became heavily involved with an outbreak of severe jaundice at Castries, St Lucia (*see* Chapter 4). Was it simply malignant malaria (*P. falciparum* infection) or **yellow fever**? His careful observations initially supported the former diagnosis, but as time passed he obtained firm evidence of the latter at post-mortem. It seems clear that *both* diseases were in fact present.

Low devoted a great deal of time to preventive strategies, i.e. eliminating swamps and breeding-sites for *mosquitoes*, an approach which had been followed by Major (later Sir Ronald) Ross (*see* Figure 8.1) in West Africa, and with whom Low corresponded (*see* below).

Only 29-years old, and with no previous experience of investigating an epidemic or implementing *preventive* strategies in practice, Low showed a remarkable degree of maturity and was clearly greatly respected by the local colonial and military authorities, despite the fact that the editor (McHugh) of the *Voice of St Lucia* (*see* Chapters 3 and 5) remained antagonistic to his endeavours.

Yellow fever in the Caribbean

Yellow fever had of course in the past been endemic in the central Americas. For long, the UK had had major interests in the Caribbean; in the eighteenth and first half of the nineteenth centuries, she had large military establishments there, but West Indies stations were generally regarded as 'very bad stations'. In William Makepeace Thackeray's (1811–63) *Vanity Fair* (written in 1847–48), there is an example of a new governor of a West Indian island – who was not expected to survive long, **yellow fever** being so common. From 1850 onwards, however, introduction of piped water-supplies with reduction in breeding grounds of *Aëdes aegypti* mosquitoes had led to a significant decline in incidence. A General Board of Health Report for 1852 (signed by Lord Shaftesbury, Edwin Chadwick and Thomas Southwood Smith) had for example, eloquently outlined the history of **yellow fever** in this geographical location.[1]

Letter XXV

St Lucia
Dec. 14th 1901.

Dear Dr. Manson,

This is a very important letter I have to write you. From above you will see I am in St. Lucia, and from what I have heard it is a good thing I am. Briefly then I got back to Barbados Saturday at noon, 2 hours after a telegram from Sir Robert Llewelyn[2] from St. Lucia came urging me to come to the **yellow fever** epidemic and the military authorities in Barbados also asked me. I wired back [that I] would come, and on Monday had an interview with the General and his staff. I said there was no doubt about the fact that the Morne [situated on a plateau about one mile above Castries – *see* Chapters 3 and 4] must be packed with *mosquitos* and that if they would give me a free hand to act as I thought fit I would be only too delighted to go and stamp out the disease and kill off all [the] *mosquitos*. Everyone was very frightened so they accepted my offer at once and I sailed the same afternoon and here I am.

Well I think apart from the **yellow fever** it was a good thing I did come. To explain I saw Gray [*see* Letter I] the 2nd day here and in talking he said he had had a letter from Ross[3] [*see* Figure 8.1] asking him to write something on the **malaria** of the place. Ross then said he would incorporate this in his reports and would send a man to St. Lucia to destroy *mosquitos* (a thing I have been [aiming] at, and doing for the last 6 months). I did not think Ross would leave this part of the world alone for long especially as he knew that I representing the London School [LSTM], was out here and I see through his little game perfectly. He would send someone out, boom the thing up in a big report and pose as the pioneer of *mosquito* destruction in the West Indies, just as in a report of his (I saw in Gray's house) he poses as the saviour of West Africa and gives Italians and others no credit. I think we can manage him however, and get the credit for the [LSTM]. It is a great pity that malarial

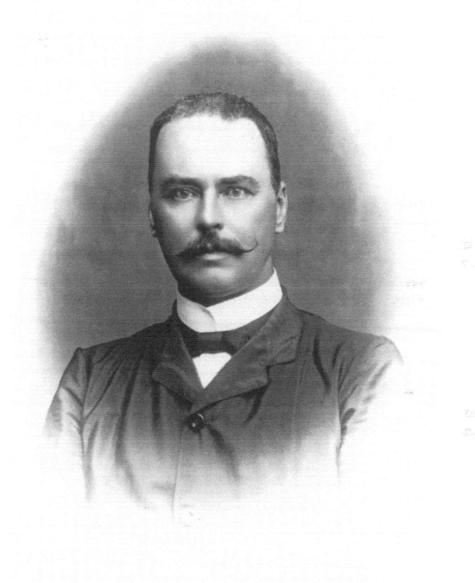

Figure 8.1: Major (later Colonel Sir) Ronald Ross FRS, KCB, KCMG (1857–1932) who, following his seminal discoveries at Secunderabad and Calcutta (Kolkata), India, was to become a leading exponent of malaria *prevention*. [*See*: G C Cook. Mosquito involvement in the malaria life cycle. *J med Biog* 1998; 6: 182–3.]

paper Gray & I wrote[4] has never appeared. Could you not get it published at once, as in it I remember advocating the destruction of *mosquitos*? That would be one stop [to] his scheme. I think next on receipt of this letter, you might put something in the medical papers, and also in the day papers about the **malarial** and **yellow fever** epidemic such as:

> Dr Low working for the [LSTM] who has been working lately at the destruction of *Culex* the filaria bearing mosquito in Barbados has proceeded to St. Lucia to enquire into the enormous epidemic of **malaria** and suspicious **yellow fever** cases that have occurred in that colony (in order to stamp out *mosquitos*). Experiments for the destruction of *anopheles* mosquitos were begun by the [LSTM] in spring in St. Lucia but want of money prevented them being carried out satisfactorily. The necessity for such has now been amply proved by the large amount of **malarial fever** now amongst the troops in St. Lucia and as the military authorities have taken the matter up we hope no expense in the way of money will be spared to completely destroy *mosquitos*. We wish the [LSTM] every success in this beneficial work and it will be interesting to see, in the light of the work being done on the West Coast of Africa by the Liverpool School of Medicine what the result will be.

I think that this should about represent the matter and get the kudos for the [LSTM]. I hate advertising myself in any way but I think after the hard work I have gone through it is only right that the London School which I represent should get the credit, and that Ross and the Liverpool people should not calmly step in and snatch up the work done.

You can see what you think of this I have just said and act accordingly, but I think it is sound & the chance I have now got as regards warring against the *mosquitos* is a magnificent one.

Well to pass to more pleasant topics than scientific jealousy. I arrived in St. Lucia at 11 AM – Tuesday, 10th, and found the place turned upside down. The steamer which I came in had to anchor at a quarantine buoy and rain descended in torrents I have seldom seen equalled. I had agreed before leaving Barbados that quarters should be found [for] me on the Morne so after seeing the administrator and Major Seton, the officer commanding the troops, I rode up the Morne, saw Major Will [and] the med officers of the station, and took up my abode just outside the end of the infected area.

What I found *was*, that sometime after building operations had begun this year in May on the Morne [a] gradually increasing epidemic of **malaria** began getting worse till in August a death occurred; October & November [there were] also a few deaths and then at the end of November 3 cases became pernicious and died with symptoms said to be typical of **yellow fever** e.g. albuminuria, black vomit &c. The civil and military doctors saw the cases, diagnosed **yellow fever** and the port was put in quarantine. The troops were then hastily removed to the [?], all building operations stopped, and this was the state of affairs when I arrived. (I append a plan of the place [which was *not* present when I had access to the correspondence] now to let you follow me more clearly.)

I had made it my [dictum] to the General & staff in Barbados before leaving, that [whether] I found the disease was only **malaria**, or was really **yellow fever** the mode of action was certain, the destruction immediately of all *mosquitos*, and I stated that I was absolutely certain I would find the Morne the infected area infested with *mosquitos*. This statement was doubted by several but as you will see I was correct.

I enquired at once on arrival for blood examinations of the cases that had died and P.M notes, but found to my disappointment that no blood tests had been accurately made and [no] P.M examinations. In this connection Gray had examined one of the cases before the suspicious ones and had found parasites, and in some of the **yellow fever** cases stated that the mononuclear leucocytes were not increased but this [is] a point that requires verification. Five cases were still in on my arrival and I went at once to see them, but they [were put] down as **yellow fever**. No 1: Woman intensely yellow full of quinine; blood exam. Nil. I suggested puncturing the spleen, but as there was opposition did not insist on it. <u>No 2 & 3:</u> Two boys in the same house mild cases of whatever they were had had, much quinine; no parasites in bl. Exam. <u>4</u>: A woman nothing definite about her at all, had had a lot of vomiting, slightly yellow, no parasites again had had much quinine. <u>5</u>: A soldier in hospital. No parasites. I made out enlarged spleen – had albuminuria 1/3 as had all the other cases in more or less amounts. I did no 5 & no 4 for leucocyte count and found 20%

and 25% of large mononuclears so if Gray is correct they were not **yellow fever**. The military Dr. thinks they are however, and in the light of their previous cases I think he is quite right to say so until it can be definitely proved. Those cases to day are all doing well & recovering so there is no chance of a P.M.

Next I inspected the Morne and found it in a state more (much more I should say) disgraceful than I expected. Building has been going on all summer, and I saw the old view of turning up the soil explained [sic] by modern methods to my hearts content and delight. At first in the dry season the many unfilled holes were all right, but when the rains came they filled with water and then later with *mosquitos*. I actually found … on this military station 800 feet above sea level, *anopheles* in millions. The people had been in the habit of digging up stones out of the ground all over the place and simply leaving the holes thus made. I counted one day 20 such holes all teaming with *anopheles*, and also found 3 imperfect drains, 2 small swamps all with *anopheles*, and dozens of old water barrels and tanks full of *C. Taeniatus* [or] the **yellow fever** mosquito. One *anopheles* pool was 50 yards from the military hospital. How on earth anyone could wonder at 50% of the troops having had fever this summer beats me entirely. The danger of turning up the soil is very clear indeed in the light of those *anopheles* infected pools. This alone I consider makes it worth my time to have come to St. Lucia.

On finding this state of affairs I at once suggested that a competent Sergeant of engineers sh. be employed and at once red tape became evident, as an order was in force that no white people were to be employed on the Morne after the **yellow fever** cases had broken out. I simply went to the Commanding Officer and asked him to telegraph to Barbados at once to have this order rescinded when required, as otherwise work was impossible and unless I had things done as I wished & suggested there was no use of me staying at all & Major Seton, officer commanding (who of course did not frame this order) was only too kind. He said he appreciated the thing at once, would take even the responsibility of ordering out white men at once, and did so. Telegraphing also to Barbados. My man a Sergeant of the R.E. [Royal Engineers] appeared this morning. I gave him a lecture on *mosquitos* took him round the ground, shewed him the larvae, and work is to begin to morrow. I got Major Will, the med. Officer, to do something officially for the order of black labourers and we will get a 100 at least [?]. Things therefore are now satisfactory and I see my way to make a splendid result out of the epidemic which should be more convincing than even the West African affair. I work from morning to night with scarcely a moments rest, and besides all this outdoor work have been going over records, books, dates of arrival of ships from infected ports to thoroughly sift the matter to the bottom to see if it is really **yellow fever** and not only very pernicious remittent [fever].

Dec. 15th.

Things are going well. A major in the R.E got fever yesterday. By blood examination I found malignant parasites and thus proved him to be a case of **malaria fever** only. This is not of course on the Morne because every white man has been cleared off except Major Will, Lieut. MacGregor, myself, and the white reduced in the hospital. The major lived at La Toe see map [*not* included with these letters].

Another man was taken ill at the same place to day. T. 104°. Blood exam. malignant rings – one pigmented, leucocytes numerous. Later, he showed undoubted pernicious symptoms and I think he is going to go like the other fatal cases e.g. he is becoming yellow, much albumin in urine and signs of suppression coming on. I hope he will get better for his own sake but still if he does die the P.M. which I have been planning already will be of the greatest importance in settling as to whether it is real **yellow fever** or only remittent [fever].

I must stop for the day as I have exhausted by [sic] news up to date but will go on again when anything turns up. I shall write [to] Ross [*see* above] a note by this mail telling him of this interesting epidemic and the steps being taken by the [LSTM] in conjunction with the Military Doctors to stop it. This I think will be useful in convincing him that we [were] in the field before him and will get us the honour for our school. I have again suggested to the administrator to have the town of Castries improved and pools filled up, a thing I did when I was here in [the] spring before.

That idiot of a man who wrote the cutting in the St. Lucia newspaper I sent you [*see* Chapter 3 and Letter XI], is on the health board and is an obstructionalist ridiculing the *mosquito* theory and objecting to have improvements done. His name is McHugh. I think you should see the Colonial Office about the whole matter. Dont say I pressed the administrator to have this done before, as he is a nice man & I do not wish to get him into trouble, but you might suggest that in view of the serious epidemic amongst the troops the town of Castries should be compelled to deal with the *mosquito* question as regards the stamping out of it, and say that as I am here I shall be very pleased to superintend and see it done thoroughly. You could mention that you have seen a cutting in a paper by a man McHugh ridiculing the thing, and have him censured or removed. It is a splendid chance and if I can help get the whip hand of them I assure you it shall be done.

I know they [?] have plenty of money and they sh. really be ordered to use some of it for the sanitation of the town. You do not need to mention that I said all this, but I know with your influence at the Col. Office you could probably have it done, as of themselves they are too supine to move.

Dec. 18th.
The case of the Captain I told you off [sic] when last I wrote was very sad. Then I think I told you I did not think he would live, and as expected he died on Monday morning suddenly. He had almost complete suppression of urine all Sunday with a lot of albuminuria and though the T° fell next morning, he could not pull through. His body was brought up to the Morne and at the P.M. it was found he had sclerosis of the mitral valve, atheroma of the aorta, subacute nephritis and **malarial fever**, his spleen having plenty [of] recent pigment and some parasites. It was therefore a pernicious malignant fever complicated by the heart condition. He was buried in the afternoon, the 2 military doctors, myself and 4 orderlies being the only people present, as he was interred in the cemetery on the Morne which is in the infected area beside the graves of the other victims.

Since that date things have been very quiet, the 4 suspected cases [of **yellow fever**] are all convalescent, and no further ones have appeared. I have been busy getting up all the details of the old cases to see where the infection came from, and so far I have not been very successful, because though some ships did come from Rio Janeiro [Brazil] an infected port, I cannot find that any of the people who died had ever been near them.

The two military doctors and myself live together and no one comes to see us, as everyone is in a state of terror in case they get infected. We are just outside the cordon but I spend all my time in the area trying to ferret things out, looking at drains & buildings &c. taking care of course not to be bitten by *mosquitos*. The drainage & filling up [of] holes is going on very satisfactorily and already there must be an enormous diminution in the *mosquito* world up there. The house we live in has no *mosquitos* as Major Will has seen to all the water tanks & barrels and other collections of water. By the way he was in Hong Kong when you were there, and he said he had met you there. We have been clearing the bush all round the place to day, and yesterday I went to [?] where the troops are now, and had a look about finding an *anopheles* pool and other things. They are busy however filling up all the holes there with sand and if the [?] would only take the matter up things would be very good indeed.

I saw the Governor [Hodgson] when in Barbados and suggested my plan of lecturing to the Sanitary Inspectors on *mosquitos*; he thought it was a very good idea and said he would make the arrangements for it but owing to this, now I don't know when I shall get there. They want me in Antigua also I have heard so I have plenty to do. I do not know where I shall partake of my Christmas dinner this year; do you remember I left your country house[5] that afternoon last year.

The quarantine should soon be raised now and then one will be able to get about a bit and leave the island when one wishes.

I have never had time to visit my old haunt Gros Islet, for the *F. Demarquaii* [sic] yet but will do so some day soon when I have time. I must stop now as I have exhausted my news.

So with best wishes to you all at Queen Anne Street for a happy New Year.

Believe me.
Yours sincerely
G. C. Low.

P.S.
I shall add anything of importance to morrow if such happens.
G.L.
Address. Bay Mansions, Barbados still they know where to forward my letters.

Letter XXVI

The Morne
St Lucia
Jan. 03. 02.

Dear Dr. Manson,

I am still here, and developments have taken place since last mail i.e. I am now certain that the disease here has been real **yellow fever**,[6] a case having appeared last week. Briefly then a Capt. Despard took ill suddenly, I examined his blood at once & found no parasites. After that he had quinine, but did not respond; he quickly got albuminous urine, severe vomiting, and other symptoms, and passed into the typhoid state with low muttering delirium, becoming very yellow all over. Even then all the symptoms would have answered to a pernicious **malaria** fever. He gradually sank & died. I got a P.M. a few hours after death, and then in conjunction with Major Will [*see* above] and the other army medical men found the following: Yellow liver fatty degeneration. Spleen almost normal in size and colour & appearance, no pigmentation, not malarial. Kidneys, congestion probably early nephritis. Brain some congestion. Miscroscop. all organs no parasites; not a speck of malaria pigment. There was not a trace of **malaria** about the thing and I forgot to say the stomach had the black coffee ground fluid so typical of **yellow fever** in it. There is no doubt it was **Y. fever** and the case was then returned as such.

I thought the thing was over but I fear more cases will now crop up, as this one was a long way distant from where the original ones came from. The island has been quarantined again of course and there is great excitement amongst the shop keepers and coal merchants, as steamers will not come to coal here, and trade suffers. The onus of their excitement and wrath, for what reason I cant say, has fallen upon me. Some little shop and store keepers I believe got up a deputation protesting against the diagnosis of **yellow fever**, but as the brains of such individuals are incompetent to judge on such matters they have not made much impression on any of the educated people about. You have no idea of the difficulties that beset one in these parts.

Our friend Galgay [sic] [*see* Letter I] has come out in quite a new light. I told you he was a cantankerous ass before, but now he really has excelled all his previous attainments. In the early cases of **yellow fever** he and Gray examined the blood for parasites, the latter found none the former found the blood full of spores! and flagellae! and therefore came to the conclusion the case was **malaria**. They had been called in to consult with the military people. Everyone at that time decided the cases were **yellow fever** but Galgey posing I think as a martyr, and more for his pecuniary emoluments persisted against everyone. The value of his blood examinations you will appreciate from the spores and flagellae, the former of those he having mistaken for bacilli according to Major Will who saw the specimen.

I had to wait some time you see before I could get a case on which to decide but at last it came with the result I have already mentioned. After the administrator was told about the result he suggested that the 3 civilian doctors should come and have a meeting with the military doctors and myself who should give them the full notes and details of the case. This was done. Dennehy & Gray [*see* Chapter 4] were unanimous in upholding the diagnosis, but Galgey though he admitted there was not the slightest evidence of **malaria** still insisted the case was one of **malaria**. He has now become so silly that no one pays the slightest attention to him, and he may be left out [of] further consideration.

I fear as I said before further cases will be certain to occur and at present there are 2 exceedingly suspicious mild cases. They are not cases of **malaria** from the blood exam, and [not] **typhoid** or other fever [but] it is evident there are good grounds for suspicion.

The destruction of *mosquitos* is going on apace. I can't now find a single *anopheles* in the Morne, all pools have been filled and the drains and swampy bits cleaned out. The rain water tanks have caused a good lot of trouble, many being full of *C. taeniatus* [and] our friend of **yellow fever**. However the military authorities have done very well and if only the town would do the same there would be few *mosquitos* left. Don't forget our obstructionist friend Mr. McHugh, creatures like him only encumber the earth and cause no end of trouble by the emanations poured out from their empty skulls.

The introduction of the fever must undoubtedly have resulted from infected *mosquitos* being brought in steamers from Rio and other ports. There is a big trade with steamers from those ports coming to coal here, and after 14 days they lie alongside the wharf. It is therefore very simple for our friend to find his way ashore and bite susceptible persons. There are many very interesting points still requiring looking into however as regards the exact aetiology [and] of its spread by *C. taeniatus*.

I have been so busy lately in the work of destroying *mosquitos* that I have not had time to look Gros Islet and the Filaria *Demarquaii* [sic] up, but I hope if things quiet[en] down I shall get a chance. As soon as I can get out of St. Lucia I shall go to St. Kitts finish it, then off for my big mosq. campaign to Barbados.

With best regards to Mrs. Manson & yourself.

Believe me &c.

G. C. Low

A letter to Manson from Low's father

A letter dated 19 January 1902 (Letter XXVII) is to be found amongst those from Low to Manson and was written by Low's father – S M Low (*see* Appendix 1). In it he thanks Manson for continuing assistance to his son; the reason(s) for his writing at this time remains unclear, but seems to relate to a loan of the above letters (for 1901) for perusal. It is possible, though evidence is lacking, that Manson, realising that Low's life was in potential danger – due to his exposure to **yellow fever** cases – felt compelled to encourage access to this correspondence.

Letter XXVIII

St Lucia
Jan. 27. 02.

Dear Dr. Manson,

I expected a letter from you last mail, but as my letters have been coming very irregularly lately I expect it has missed me, probably gone to some of the other islands. I had a letter from Major Ross [*see* Letter XXV] last mail in reply to a note I sent him, and he also sent me his report on the West Coast,[7] and some statistics on the **yellow fever** in Cuba.[8] The results of those especially the latter are truly marvellous. I don't think he knew that I had been working at the destruction of *mosquitos* here and his letter was very nice.

The **yellow fever** is now completely dead and we have completely destroyed the *mosquitos* on the Morne where it broke out. This was comparatively simple, drainage doing away with the *anopheles*, and fumigation and making the roofs of the water tanks *mosquito* proof doing the same for the *culex*. The condition of affairs is therefore good. Negie [?] the other military place is still having **malarial fever** but the large swamp is now filled up and it is decreasing undoubtedly. The town has not done much and they must be stimulated from home.

That ass of a newspaper man [*see* Letter XXVI] is still writing idiotic articles in his paper and I wish you could do something to stop him. Work has been fairly brisk lately with some of the malarial cases. I had a very nice P.M. examination of one, and got beautiful parasites in the spleen and other internal organs.

I heard from Daniels [*see* Letter VIII] and from Theobald [*see* Letter IV] last mail. The latter gave me an account of some of the *mosquitos* from B Guiana. I must have found a tremendous number of new ones.

I go back to Barbados on Friday. I shall lay a programme before the Governor [Hodgson], and start lectures to the Sanitary Authorities on *mosquitos*. I then hope a certain number of men will be detailed off to form a *mosquito* brigade e.g. to fill up wells and otherwise destroy larvae. You have no idea how much opposition one meets with amongst the public on such subjects; most of them treat the matter in an inert way while others however actually oppose it. Another class believe it are very interested but do nothing after all that is suggested. However I have hopes of Barbados as the place is more civilised than St. Lucia and I shall strive to din it into them.

I had a letter from Dr Ozzard[9] the other day. I sent him a paper on Filarial lymphangitis[10] for the *British Guiana annual* [author's italics] which he is trying to start again. I illustrated it with some cases and charts, and put in some little new points. He wants me to go back there I believe, but the chance of stamping out *mosquitos* there is rather remote. The whole point really turns on the money. If one has that it is simple but the colonies are hard to move to spend any of their own. I have been getting parasites in animal blood lately, plenty [?] in pigeons. Bats are difficult to get. I have no[t] had much time for filaria lately but hope to get some more cases, especially P.Ms, in Barbados.

I wonder if Dr. Morris went to see you … when in London.

I must stop for the present but will go again the day after tomorrow if anything fresh turns up.

Believe me

Yours sincerely

G. C. Low

Thursday

30th. Jan. 02.

I have not much to add in the way of news. I go to Barbados to morrow. I saw Gray yesterday. He hopes to get something in Sierra Leone he says [*see* Letter V]. Galgey I also saw. He had nothing fresh and said he had no trace of *F. Demarquaii* [sic]. He has his hand on no other cases at present, so will not likely get fresh adults.

Ross I see had taken the trouble to write [to] McHugh the editor of the paper I have spoken of. I saw an edition yesterday full of another absurd and very unjust article, blaming Gray and telling several absolute lies about myself. I don't think it worth worry however, If you can reach him at the Colonial Office do so by all means.

I hope to hear from you this next mail and I should get your letter on Monday at Barbados. I am sure Sir F. Hodgson [*see* Chapter 5] will lend all support in that island as he is very keen on the thing.

What do you think of the man who found the 3 new malarial parasites in the trop. journal lately?[11] His technique to start with was fallacious and I expect he saw specks of stain and dirt. The men who found parasites in all the cases in hospital in Hong Kong must evidently [have] been looking at vacuoles at least it does not hold good for here or any other tropical place I have been in. I must stop now as I have nothing more to say.

With best regards.

Believe me.

Yrs Sincerely

G. C. Low

P.S.

I hear Theobald's monograph on the *mosquito*[12] is out. I don't know if the museum will send me a copy, but if not, you might get one for me and I shall pay for it when I come home. I believe there are 3 volumes. Could you have it sent by next mail.

G. C. Low

References and Notes

1 Shaftesbury, E Chadwick, T Southward Smith. *General Board of Health: second report on quarantine: Yellow fever*. London: H M Stationery Office. 1852: 414.

2 **Sir Robert Baxter Llewelyn** KCMG (1845–1919) was Governor of the Windward Islands (1900–06). He had previously served in Jamaica, Tobago and St Vincent; from 1891–1900 he was Administrator of the Colony of the Gambia. [*See also*: Anonymous. Llewellyn, Sir Robert Baxter. *Who Was Who 1916–1928*. 5th ed. London: A & C Black 1992: 491.]

3 **Major (later Colonel Sir) Ronald Ross**, was Professor of Tropical Medicine at the Liverpool School of Tropical Medicine. He had documented the life-cycle of *Proteosoma* sp in avian malaria in India at Calcutta (Kolkata) in 1898. W F Bynum. Ross, Sir Ronald (1857–1932). In: H C G Matthew, B Harrison (eds). *Oxford Dictionary of National Biography*. Oxford: Oxford University Press 2004; 47: 842–6. [*See also*: Anonymous. Ross, Colonel Sir Ronald. *Who Was Who, 1929–1940*. 2nd ed. London: A & C Black 1967: 1172.]

4 St. G Gray, G C Low. Malarial fever in St Lucia, W.I. *Br med J* 1902; i: 193–4.

5 Manson then had a country house at Chalfont St Giles, Buckinghamshire which he had purchased in 1897. (P H Manson-Bahr, A Alcock. *The life and work of Sir Patrick Manson*. London: Cassell and Co Ltd 1927: 117.)

6 This prompted Low to write an article on the diagnostic differences between yellow fever and severe *Plasmodium falciparum* infection (*see* Chapter 10). [*See also*: G C Low. The differential diagnosis of yellow fever and malignant malaria. *B med J* 1902; ii: 860–1; G Williams. *The Plague Killers*. New York: Charles Scribner's Sons 1969: 345.]

7 H E Annett, J E Dutton, J H Elliott. *Report of the Malaria Expedition to Nigeria of the Liverpool School of Tropical Medicine and Medical Parasitology*. Liverpool: University Press of Liverpool 1901: 68; J E Dutton, F V Theobald. *Report of the Malaria Expedition to the Gambia 1902*. London: The University Press of Liverpool 1903: 46. [*See also*: R Ross. *Malarial Fever: its cause, prevention, and treatment*. London: Longmans, Green & Co 1902 (new ed.): 68; R Ross. *Mosquito brigades and how to organise them*. London: George Philip & Son 1902: 98; R Ross. *Observations on malaria by Medical Officers of the Army and others*. London: H M Stationery Office 1919: 342.]

8 G C Cook. *Tropical Medicine: an illustrated history of the pioneers*. London: Academic Press 2007: 103–13.

9 Albert Tronson Ozzard – *see* Preface. [*See also*: D I Grove. *A History of Human Helminthology*. Wallingford, Oxon: CAB International 1990: 812–3.]

10 G C Low. Filarial lymphangitis. *J trop Med* 1902; 5: 255–6. [*See also*: B. *Guiana Med Ann* 1902; 14: 1–9.]

11 *See* G Thin. The etiology of malarial fever. *J trop Med* 1899: 1–6.

12 F V Theobald. *A monograph of the culicidae or mosquitoes. Mainly compiled from the collections received at the British Museum from various parts of the world in connection with the investigation into the cause of malaria conducted by the Colonial Office and The Royal Society*. London: British Museum (Natural History) 1901: 37 plates. Theobald also wrote three other monographs on mosquitoes about this time.

Chapter 9

St Kitts, and the voyage to London (February–April 1902)

The final phase of Low's expedition concentrated largely on mosquito-*control*. This had now become his major interest, and he obviously intended making a mark for the LSTM in the Caribbean in the same way that Ross (*see* Chapter 8) had done in West Africa. Finally, after some 15 months, he was summoned home 'as soon as possible' by Manson – presumably in order to prepare him for the 'sleeping sickness' expedition to Uganda.[1] In view of his 'obsession' with filariae, together with his London observations, Manson clearly favoured *Filaria (Mansonella) perstans* as the likely candidate as the *cause* of the 'negro lethargy'.

Letter XXIX

Bay Mansion
Barbados
Feb. 15. 02.

Dear Dr. Manson,
This is mail morning and I have been so busy I have not had time to start my letter before this. I shall therefore have time only for a short note. Things have been going well. First, I got your letter the day after I got back to Barbados. Thanks very much for it. I at once wrote a report on the **yellow fever** epidemic and sent it with a covering letter to Sir Robert Llewelyn [*see* Letter XXV] … Governor of the Windward Islands in which St. Lucia is incorporated. The General commanding the troops with whom I had a long talk on coming back from St. Lucia asked for a copy of it, and as it dealt largely with the military side of the matter I gave him a copy stating it to be so and saying that the original had been sent to the Governor of the Windward Islands for transmission home, in a covering letter. I suppose this is all right and the Colonial Office wont mind.

I saw the Governor Sir F. Hodgson [*see* Chapter 5] on arrival and made arrangements for giving the Sanitary Inspectors a series of lectures on the destruction of *mosquitos*. He made all the arrangements very kindly and said he would do everything in his power. I gave the first lecture last Friday a sample of which I send you to day and another yesterday. I shall send it [to] you by next mail, and my next one. You might if you think it worth while give them to the tropical journal for publication. They would I think be useful for other places to follow out the suggestions, and it would show our Liverpool friends that London is 'also working' at the *mosquito* question. I go round with the Sanitary Inspectors in person and point out what should be done and I have early hopes that a great improvement in the *mosquitos* should take place. It is only however by constantly pegging at them that one will get results as the people require a lot of education still on the subject, and a lot are very lethargic. Still with the Government backing me it makes the matter simpler as I think I shall persuade them to pass laws on the question of standing water.

The Government here are printing 100 copies of each for distribution, and I think it would do no harm sending some to the other islands. You will see the report on St. Lucia when the Colonial Office get it; I have put the facts plainly and have not spared the town of Castries as I really think its condition is disgraceful, and if white troops are to be placed in St. Lucia the place must first be rendered fit for them living in. However you will read it for yourself and see what you think of it, and then the action the Colonial Office will take up will depend on it. The military authorities have behaved splendidly and have paid for all the work done when I was there & have got a fresh grant of money I believe to carry on further improvements.

I am busy cutting sections of tissues from St. Lucia at present and have been going hard at **filarial cases** here lately, there have [been] some very good ones clinically.

I shall not get to St. Kitts this mail as I expected, as it is better to finish my lectures here and press on [with] the *mosquito* hygiene. If I broke them by leaving in the middle they would have forgotten about them before I come back again. However I shall do it later.

I see the mail from St. Lucia this morning is flying the quarantine flag & have just heard there is a suspicious case on board. I should think it will be probably a malarial case and I expect they will ask me to look at it. A blood examination should decide.

I have no more time for now. So with best regards to all at Queen Anne Street.

Believe me
Yours sincerely
G. C. Low

Letter XXX

Bay Mansion
Barbados
Feb. 28. 02.

My dear Dr. Manson,

Having finished Barbados for a time I go to St. Kitts on Monday to see what there is in that island. I finished my lectures here this week and send you in a separate envelope my second and third. What I have done is, given these lectures, shewn the people specimens, and have personally visited with the Sanitary Inspectors different parts of the town pointing out to them what is wrong & what is required. I have also put in a suggestion to the Governor [Hodgson] to have a law passed about standing water. Having done all this it now really rests with them to carry out the reforms themselves so I cant do much more. I shall therefore … do St. Kitts in the next fortnight and then come back and see how things are getting on here. I shall again go with the Inspectors and press on the passing of the law about the water if that is not already done.

What do you think I should do after that? Do you think I should come home and go to the West Coast to Lagos say, or Mauritius the latter place being unhealthy would give good scope for hygienic improvements. Write and say what you think. As the time is going on I should like to have a try at the host of *perstans*. We had a case of **small pox** here the other day and it is quite likely it may spread and if it does it will be a very severe epidemic as few of the inhabitants are vaccinated.[2] I have been getting some more interesting **filaria** cases, and I have been cutting sections of material I got in St. Lucia …. There has been no fresh outbreak [of **yellow fever**] in St. Lucia and things are apparently prospering there at present, though the

malarial fever still is rampant. I dont expect to find very much in St. Kitts; there is a good lot of filarial disease but not much **malaria** I believe.

I saw a Dr. from Trinidad and one from Demerara [British Guiana] the other day. Both were on their way home for a course at the Tropical School. I hear from Dr Ozzard [*see* Preface] every now and again and I sent him a paper for their *medical annual* [author's italics] which they are going to start again. I got Noe's [?] paper all right, I cant translate it perfectly but it seems to be hostile I think.

With best regards
Believe me
Yours sincerely
G. C. Low

Letter XXXI

Basseterre
St. Kitts
March. 11. 02.

My dear Dr. Manson,

I have just concluded my visit to St. Kitts and it has been a very enjoyable and successful one the people having taken such a very keen interest in everything I have done.

Briefly then there is a minimum of **malaria** due to a small swamp near the [major] town but **filarial disease** is rampant, no fewer than 32% of the people having it. It is the most heavily infected island I have yet done and I have seen some splendid cases here. Viz. pedunculated groin **elephantiasis**, elephantiasis of the arms, all sorts in the legs and some huge scrotums. [?] people of the best classes have come to be examined quite readily, and 6 out of 20 had it, they being infected I should say quite as frequently as the negro, as I have heard of many others with developed symptoms. It beats Barbados hollow, though it is bad enough there. I got 2 cases of *Demarquaii* [sic], one in a man who has been in Dominica the other in a Portuguese who came, and a young man who has only been out of the island once [to] Port of Spain, Trinidad, since coming. He, I think, must have got it in St. Kitts so that makes another island where it is found.

The people of this island as I said have been the most enthusiastic of any of the other islands and they have driven me all over the place and so I have got no end of work done in the time spent here. I gave a lecture last night at which over 200 people were present and they followed it with great interest and I am sure believe in the *mosquito* now.

On getting back to Barbados where I start for to morrow morning I shall write the Administrator a report on what they will have to do to put down their **filarial disease**. Their malarial swamp is simple, and the filaria business is also easy as they have a pipe water supply. Their privies [are] filthy pits dug in the ground [and] are the chief breeding grounds of the *culex* and I shall get them to abolish those altogether. I think after my lecture they will all sleep under *mosquito* nets so in a very short time an enormous improvement may be hoped for. After the lethargy and hostility of the people of St. Lucia it is quite a treat to meet with an intelligent and pleasant community like this.

As I say I go back to Barbados to morrow and I shall see the Governor [Hodgson] and press on [with] the work there. They must go on with it themselves now as I really cant do much more that [sic] I have done but I shall again personally take the Sanitary Inspectors round and shew them the places.

On receipt of this letter you might write me and say what you think I should do now. This will reach you about the end of March and the reply will get [to] me about the middle or end of April i.e. just at the end of my two years. I should like very much to have a go at Africa to try for *filaria perstans* and its host.[3] Say if you think I should come home and go out there or if I sh. stay out in the West Indies for some time longer. Of course even if I got home as late as September to England I would still have time for some months on the West Coast before my last year would be up. I have pretty well worked up the W. Indies now [the] only thing missing being that intermediate host of *F. Demarquaii* [sic]. That must be an insect, as I told you I had seen the sausage stage in *C. taeniatus* once or twice but never further. If we could find the host of *perstans* it would give a good clue to *Demarquaii* [sic].

I shall go on doing as much work as I can till I get your reply, and then we can see what is to be done.

Lagos would be a good place as I know they have *perstans* at

Ibadan in the interior where Dr. Rice[4] is, and Sir W. McGregor[5] would give every facility I am sure. However write me and say what you advise.

I was sorry to hear from your letter that you had had such a nasty attack of gout but I hope by now you are better. I had a relapse of my [malarial] fever the other day in Barbados, an exact miniature of the first go, lasting for two days or so. Quinine quickly cured it however and my health keeps good.

We had a wire here this morning about Lord Methuen[6] being caught by the Boers.[7] It is a great pity as it will spoil the termination of the war.

I have a three days journey before me from here to Barbados, going with the steamer that takes this letter home.

I must stop now as I am very busy and have no more time.

With best regards to Mrs. Manson and yourself.

Believe me.

Yours sincerely

G. C. Low

Letter XXXII

Bay Mansion

Barbados

Ap. 2. 02.

Dear Dr. Manson,

I got your letter per mail about coming home as soon as possible [in order to proceed to Uganda]. After enquiring about it I have decided to leave the West Indies on April the 12th. arriving in London about April the 24th. The following mail after that was full & could not take me, and as the **small pox** has caused quarantine for Halifax [Nova Scotia, Canada] I find they will not take me that way either. This is practically then my only chance for some time so I have taken it. My work here is finished, and I cannot get to any other island as they have all quarantined Barbados. I dont know if the **smallpox** is to spread soon or not but I hope now it waits till I get clear of the place.

I send this via New York in the hopes it will get home before I do myself. If it does not you shall see me first. I shall just have time to finish up some things here, and I shall see about having the bloods tested annually.

With best regards.
Believe me.
Yours sincerely
G. C. Low

References and Notes

1   G C Cook. Correspondence from Dr George Carmichael Low to Dr Patrick Manson during the first Ugandan sleeping sickness expedition. *J med Biog* 1993; 1: 215–29.

2   Smallpox (variola) vaccination had been introduced by Edward Jenner (1749–1823) in 1796. However, widespread use of the vaccine took many decades to become established – especially amongst indigenous 'tropical' communities. [*See also*: D Baxby. Jenner, Edward (1749–1823). In: H C G Matthew, B Harrison (eds). *Oxford Dictionary of National Biography*. Oxford: Oxford University Press 2004; 30: 4–8.]

3   *Op cit*. See Note 1 above.

4   **Thomas Edmund Rice** was a Senior Medical Officer in southern Nigeria. He had qualified LSA from King's College, London in 1894, and was later a Medical Officer in the Gold Coast (now Ghana). [*See also*: *Medical Directory*. London: J & A Churchill 1909: 1614.]

5   **Sir William MacGregor** MD GCMG (1846–1919) at that time Governor of Lagos, was a great colonial administrator. Himself an Aberdeen medical graduate he formed a close relationship with Ross in preventive strategies in West Africa. [*See also:* Anonymous. MacGregor, Rt. Hon. Sir William. *Who Was Who 1916–1928*. 5th ed. London: A & C Black 1992: 517; F P Sprent, L Milne. MacGregor, Sir William (1846–1919). In: H C G Matthew, B Harrison (eds). *Oxford Dictionary of National Biography*. Oxford: Oxford University Press 2004; 35: 444–5.]

6   **Field-Marshal Paul Sanford Methuen** GCB, GCMG, GCVO (1845–1932) (third Baron). This reference is to the battle at Tweebosch [*see*: T Pakenham. *The Scramble for Africa*. Abacus 1992.] [*See also*: Anonymous. Methuen, 3rd Baron, Field Marshal Paul Sanford Methuen. *Who Was Who 1929–1940*. 2nd ed. London: A & C Black 1967: 935; C T Atkinson, R T Stearn. Methuen, Paul Sanford, third Baron Methuen (1845–1932). In: H C G Matthew, B Harrison (eds). *Oxford Dictionary of National Biography*. Oxford: Oxford University Press 2004; 37: 968–9.] Methuen was also severely wounded in this battle.

7   The South African (or Boer) Wars took place between October 1899 and May 1902. Methuen was, at the time of his capture, Commander of the First Division of the First Army Corps in South Africa.

Chapter 10

Contributions of Low's Caribbean expedition to scientific knowledge and disease prevention

Chapters 4–9 consist of transcriptions of 31 letters sent by Low to his mentor (Manson) in London. During a fifteen-month period he had thus accumulated a vast amount of factual information. Although he had written several 'papers' during his travels, much remained to be submitted for publication, and this chapter concentrates on Low's *published* work which emanated from the Caribbean expedition. Although today, the cause and ideal preventive strategies for lymphatic filariasis, malaria and yellow fever are well known to all and sundry, in 1901–02 relevant facts were still at an early and experimental stage, and existing knowledge was geographically localised.

Malaria prevalence in St Lucia

The reader should appreciate that Ross's discoveries in India had taken place in 1897 and 1898, a relatively short time before Low's expedition of 1901–02.

A joint paper (his first from the Caribbean), with St George Gray, consisted of an analysis of data obtained from a large number of 'native' patients with malaria infection who had visited the Castries and district dispensaries for treatment between 14 January and 4 April 1901 (the months of maximal transmission in St Lucia). Blood films from 230 cases were examined (in the wet state); 137 (none of whom had received quinine) were infected with *Plasmodium* spp. Table 10.1 summarises the results. 'As age advances,' the authors concluded, 'the percentage of infections [still] remains high, and there does not seem to be any very marked immunity attained.' This, they considered, provided evidence that 'the West Indian negro differs from his African ancestors in his susceptibility to malarial fever'. They clearly found this fact difficult to explain:

Table 10.1: Results of Low's (joint) paper on malaria prevalence in St Lucia*

	Children				
	< 2 years	2–9 years	10–20 years	≥ 21 years	TOTAL
Number of cases seen at dispensary	87	174	260	544	1,065
Number of cases examined	49	71	60	50	230
Number of cases infected with *Plasmodium* spp	22	46	38	31	137
Malignant parasites alone	14	32	24	19	89 ⎫
Malignant parasites with crescents	2	5	7	6	20 ⎬ 109
Benign tertian parasites	3	1	5	3	12
Quartan parasites	–	1	1	–	2
Double infections†	2	3	–	1	6
Pigmented leucocytes alone	1	4	1	2	8
Not infected	27	25	22	19	93

* St G Gray, G C Low. *Br med J* 1902; i: 193–4.
† Malignant and benign tertian.

It is a well-known fact that natives when brought to a new part of the tropics from their original home, suffer severely from the fever of the district: but then the West Indian is not a recent importation; he has lived now for a considerable time in those islands, and has become thoroughly acclimatised to the climate and customs of his new home. One must remember, however, that he is no longer a savage; he is semi-civilised, wears clothes, and more or less lives the same life as the white residents. Further, in the West Indian the question of a mixed race must always be considered. In St. Lucia there is a very large coloured population, varying greatly in degree, the result of interbreeding between white and black; many of the cases treated at the dispensaries were of this mixed class.

Clinical presentation in those infected with *P falciparum* was then described:

> In … malignant cases the symptoms varied greatly in severity, 8 showing pernicious complications. Two of those were moribund when brought to the dispensary, and both died within a few hours after being seen. One collapsed exhibiting the algid type of the disease, the other in a state of complete coma. Both received hypodermic injections of quinine as soon as the examination of the blood showed [*P falciparum*], but the disease was too far advanced for this to be of any use. The after-history of the remaining 6 is unknown, as the patients refused to go to hospital and returned to their homes in the country. No cases of hyperpyrexia were seen.

Observations made to determine various entomological aspects of malaria in and around Castries were then described in detail:

> Wherever possible the neighbourhood of the dwelling-houses of people suffering from malarial fever was explored with a view to finding the breeding places of *Anopheles*, and in every case such search was successful. The common *Anopheles* of St. Lucia is the *Anopheles albipes* (Theobald), easily recognised by its spotted wings and its characteristic white hind tarsi. It is not a domestic mosquito, never having been found in dwelling-houses during the day; it probably hides in mango trees, bushes, or cane fields in the vicinity. Though never seen in a state of nature by day, insects imprisoned in test tubes will bite readily at any time.
>
> The larvae are found in large numbers in all the valleys and low-lying parts of the island. As a rule one river descends through each valley, and at this season of the year, when there is little water in them, the surf beating on the shore completely blocks up their mouths. As a result a stagnant lagoon is formed behind this barrier, and in those larvae were found in tremendous numbers. The villages of the island are situated on the seashore at the mouths of those valleys – generally within a few yards of the rivers – so the prevalence of the malarial fever in them is easily explained. Round the town of Castries the conditions are different. The Castries River comes

down behind the town and opens into the harbour, but, except in the rainy season, it is very sluggish, and numerous small backwaters covered with vegetation exist along its banks; in those the mosquito deposits her eggs and the larvae develop. Unfortunately native houses are crowded along its bank, and the cases of fever from Castries examined at the dispensary mostly all come from this infected area.

Anopheles larvae were also found in a small river course to the north of the town, in an open drain in the immediate vicinity of the town, and in pools of stagnant water adjacent to the Botanical Gardens. The mountainous parts of the island are more or less free from larvae, though in January, 1901, they were found at a height of nearly 800 feet at the back of Morne Fortune, one of the hills behind the town of Castries. This species of mosquito was also found in Dominica, close to the town of Roseau, breeding in an irrigated cane-field, and also in a backwater of the main river; near those areas malarial fever existed. Amongst a series of mosquitos sent by Mr. Lefroy from Antigua *A. albipes* was again present, so it is extremely probable that it is the common *Anopheles* of most of the West Indian Islands.

Preventive strategies for malaria

However, a major concern of these authors was to introduce *preventive* strategies to lower the incidence of malaria in Castries:

> The prevention of malaria in the town of Castries resolves itself into a system of better drainage and sanitary improvement. The river in its course through the town ought to have its banks walled in so as to prevent sluggish accumulation of water, as was done with such beneficial results with the Tiber in Rome, and some of the smaller infected places could quite easily be drained. For Europeans residence on the slopes of the hills overlooking the town is indicated. The officers, the troops, and other people living on the Morne very rarely suffer from fever, and though cases do occur, especially amongst the soldiers, it is probable that they were infected in the town. For

people compelled to live in the town, especially in the parts near the river, the mosquito net is always indicated. The question of the valleys and other malarious parts of the island is more difficult. The mouths of the rivers could be periodically opened during the dry season to prevent as much as possible the formation of the stagnant lagoons, but as regards the swamps found in the flat parts at the north and south of the island only an extensive system of drainage would suffice.[1]

Low was greatly intrigued at the absence of mosquitoes belonging to the genus *Anopheles* in Barbados, an island only about 100 miles from St Lucia:

> In a paper on Malarial and Filarial Diseases in Barbadoes, W.I., read at the meeting of the [BMA] at Cheltenham [in] 1901, I pointed out that mosquitoes of the genus *Anopheles* were not found in that island and gave a description of a swamp situated at Worthing, a place three miles south of Bridgetown, stating as probable that, from its close similarity to infested swamps in other islands, *Anopheles* larvae might be able to exist in it. On revisiting Barbadoes [*see* Chapter 9], after an absence of two months, a careful search of this swamp and the other collections of water at different parts of the island was again made, the examination giving the same negative results as before.
>
> When leaving Barbadoes for St. Vincent, one of the adjacent islands, a plentiful supply of water was collected from the Worthing swamp and taken to St. Vincent to determine if there was anything prejudicial in the composition of this water to the life and growth of *Anopheles* larvae. The result of the experiment proves that there is not, as larvae of *Anopheles albipes*, the common West Indian *Anopheles*, taken from a swamp at Calliaqua, three miles from Kingstown, the chief town of the island, live perfectly well in it, and develop and mature satisfactorily.
>
> This indicates that it will be a very serious thing for Barbadoes if by any chance *Anopheles* mosquitos are ever introduced into the Worthing swamp; but as this place is three miles distant from the small harbour of Bridgetown and the shipping in the bay opposite it, there is not much danger of such a calamity.[2]

The absence of 'malarial fever', and the distribution of filarial disease in Barbados formed the basis for a paper also subsequently published in the *British Medical Journal* for 1902:

> The analogy between malaria and filariasis is in many ways a close and interesting one, both as far as the tropics are concerned, being very often found coexisting in the same districts and both being spread from man to man by their own special species of mosquitos. It is, therefore, interesting to be able to point to a tropical island, namely Barbadoes, in which the former is non-existent, while the latter is extremely prevalent amongst all classes of the community.
>
> The reason for the presence of the one and the absence of the other is supplied by the fact that *Anopheles* mosquitos, the definitive host of the malarial parasite, are not found in the island, whereas *Culex fatigans*, one of the suitable intermediate hosts of *filaria nocturna* [*Wuchereria bancrofti*] abounds.

Low proceeded to give a detailed description of the geographical and physical characteristics of Barbados (the most easterly of the Caribbean Islands). Both geological and climatic factors were still considered important determinants of disease prevalence (the 'germ theory' of disease was not yet widely accepted). Of 'malarial fever' he wrote:

> On arriving in Barbadoes, and talking with the medical men practising in the town and island, all were unanimous in the statement that indigenous malarial fever does not exist in the island. Cases are frequently met with in the General Hospital [but] all of these come from some of the neighbouring islands where malaria is very common. No one could point to a case which had originated in the island itself.
>
> The interesting question now arises, are any mosquitos of the genus *Anopheles* to be found in Barbadoes or not? As may be gathered from what has already been stated, the features of the island do not lend themselves very readily for the production of suitable breeding places for these insects, with the exception of the swamp at Worthing, three miles south of Bridgetown. This swamp is situated at the foot of some elevated ground quite close to the sea, with which it communicates by a canal, the exit, however, being very often blocked up with sand thrown

up by the surf. It covers a considerable area of ground and is divided up into canals and ponds with roads and paths running through it in various directions. The water, especially in the part near the outlet, is slightly brackish, and in parts it is very stagnant, smelling strongly of suphuretted hydrogen resulting from the decomposition of vegetable material. It is probably fed by springs of water, rain, and other collections which percolate from the neighbouring high ground. The surface of the water at many places is covered with algae of various sorts and other sorts of aquatic vegetation. On looking at it, it certainly appears to be a spot favourable for the development of *Anopheles* larvae, but although larvae of a species of *Culex* and those of dragon-flies and other aquatic insects were always found in abundance, no *Anopheles* larvae could be discovered.

Confirmatory evidence of this was found in the fact that people living in the vicinity never suffered from fever, but enjoyed remarkably good health. It is probable from the close similarity of this place to *Anopheles*-infested swamps in the other and neighbouring islands, that such larvae could live here perfectly well: whether they have ever been here and have died out, or whether they have never existed, is a matter of speculation.

An examination of the other swamp at the south end of the island was not very helpful, as at the time of my visit it had only filled up with water after some very heavy rain, and contained practically no algae or other vegetation; no *Anopheles* larvae were found in it, the only result of my search being a species of *Culex* in small numbers. The creek in the centre of the town is very dirty and muddy, and is really an arm of the sea fed at its upper end by rain and other waters. Several examinations produced no larvae of any sort, the water being probably too dirty for anything to live in. All the various ponds, springs, and other collections of water, though often containing plenty of suitable vegetation, gave similar results; in some, larvae of *Culex* were found, in others nothing.

Low continued:

These observations coincide with the researches of Mr. Lefroy, Entomologist to the Imperial Department of Agriculture, who has also made a systematic search for *Anopheles* larvae with negative result.

The conclusions reached, therefore, bear out that suggested by the epidemiological fact that there is no malarial fever in the island, and [goes] to prove that without mosquitos of the genus *Anopheles* no malarial fever can exist.

Lymphatic Filariasis in Barbados

Low then addressed the enormous problem of 'filarial diseases' in the island of Barbados:

> In marked contrast to the absence of malaria is the large amount of filarial disease in Barbadoes. This is not to be wondered at when one considers the extraordinary abundance of the common domestic mosquito of those parts, *Culex fatigans*, which acts as an efficient host for the spread of the disease. It is an interesting fact that out of more than 600 blood examinations of people from all parts of the island, only *filaria nocturna* [*Wuchereria bancrofti*] was found, *filaria Demarquaii* [sic], which exists in St. Vincent and St. Lucia, and which I lately found in Dominica, never being met with. Although Bridgetown has now a very good water supply, brought in pipes from the centre of the island, where it is pumped up from the subterranean collections of water, yet many tanks exist in the gardens of the large houses for watering purposes, and around the neighbouring huts barrels and tubs of water are kept and left standing for considerable times. In these situations myriads of *Culex fatigans* breed and multiply and eventually may act as propagators of the disease. An examination of the night blood of 600 cases (taken irrespectively of the patients suffering from disease or not) from the General Hospital, Central Almshouse, and from private sources, will show to what extent filariasis prevails in Barbadoes.
>
> The proportion of 14 infected whites out of 39 is manifestly much too high to be regarded as representing the degree of infection in the white population as a whole. Many of these whites for one reason or another were collected in the almshouse at the time of examination, others being more or less selected private cases.

Table 10.2 indicates the numbers of the white and 'coloured' populations affected.

> The figures referring to white people make clear a point on which sufficient evidence has not been laid before, namely, that *the white person is quite susceptible to filarial disease* [author's italics]. This is specially so as regards Barbadoes, where persons, whether resident in the island all their lives, or only visiting it temporarily, often contract the disease; the rich and poor are alike in this respect. In analysing the table [*see* Table 10.2], 27 or 4.5 per cent. of the total number examined, or 33.5 per cent. of the filarial cases, had definite pathological changes indicative of filarial disease such as elephantiasis, chyluria, filarial lymphangitis, etc.; whereas 49 of the filarial cases, or 8.1 per cent. of the total examined, had no symptoms whatever, the diagnosis being come to by the discovery of embryos [microfilariae] in the blood. This latter class is a dangerous one as regards the spread of the disease, for it is manifest that unless sleeping under mosquito nets, which if they are negroes they never do, they nightly infect many mosquitos, which in turn infect other people and so spread the disease.
>
> To get some idea of the number of infected mosquitos about, a series of dissections of 100 mosquitos, of the species *Culex fatigans* taken from the wards and corridors of the General Hospital, in which there were cases with embryos circulating in their blood was carried out. Of this number, 23 per cent. were

Table 10.2: Prevalence of *Filaria nocturna* infection in different ethnic groups in Barbadoes*

Race [ethnic group]	Number investigated	Non-infected	Infected
Negroes	401	357	44
Mulattos	160	142	18
Whites	39	25	14
TOTAL	600	524	76[†]

* G C Low. *Br med J* 1902; i: 1472–3.
† Overall 12.66%.

found to be infected with *filaria nocturna* [*Wuchereria bancrofti*] at various stages of development, and in one mature forms were found in the proboscis, thus showing the danger of being near infected people.

Preventive strategies for lymphatic filariasis

The question arises, What can be done for the *prevention* [author's italics] of filarial disease? Much has now been done and tried for the destruction of *Anopheles*, the malaria-bearing mosquito. Similar or modified methods should be carried out for all domestic mosquitos. Considering that their breeding places are confined to houses and their vicinity, this should not prove a task at all approaching in magnitude to the draining of large swamps or to treating them in other ways.

Taking Barbadoes as an example, as has already been stated, there is now a perfect water supply, and people can get their water fresh from the standpipes at their doors. Such being the case, old wells ought to be filled up; no water barrels or tubs should be allowed, or if kept they should be emptied every week or so. Tanks and collections of water in gardens should all be periodically treated with kerosene or be furnished with closely-fitting covers to prevent mosquitos getting in.

These methods are simple and inexpensive, and each householder should see that they are applied in his garden and grounds. The difficulty begins when one has to take into account the inability of the negro to grasp anything of a hygienic nature. The only way to get over this would be a system of sanitary inspection by a few competent men. For individual prophylaxis *mosquito* nets ought always to be used, but many, even educated, people still persist in sleeping without them; of course nothing in this line can be expected of the native population.

If such means were adopted for Barbadoes, the prevalence of filarial disease, which is at present quite alarming, could easily, with little trouble and expense, be greatly diminished, and thus save much suffering, as well as loss of time, hideous deformity, and doubtless, in not a few instances, loss of life.[3]

This report again emphasised the fact that *prevention* was very much to the forefront of Low's mind at this time; this was perhaps more in line with the philosophy and policy of the Liverpool rather than the LSTM.

Filaria demarquayi

A further conclusion to emerge from Low's Caribbean expedition is his dogged perseverance in attempting to master any situation, or solve a specific problem. This is exemplified by his intensive search for the host of *Filaria demarquayi*. He began a paper summarising his observations with a brief history and description of the 'embryos' (microfilariae) of this organism and continued with careful epidemiological details, in which prevalence of the organism in the various islands came to the fore:

> *St Lucia.* – Out of a total of 472 persons examined from all parts of the island, 23, or 4.87 per cent., were found to be infected with embryos of *filaria Demarquaii* [sic], but a detailed examination of the special districts infected brought out the interesting fact that the parasite was very limited in its distribution; 16 of the 23 cases came from Gros Islet, a native village in the north part of the island, situated on sandy soil on the sea coast, with swampy ground and scrub bush around it. Of the other 7 infected cases, 2 had lived on Gros Islet, 1 near it, another at Monchy, also a village on the north coast, while the remaining 3 had never been in that part of the island having lived in or about Castries, the main town. Soufriere, the second town of the island, and Vieux Fort, a village at the south of the island, always gave negative results. This sharp limitation of the parasite in St. Lucia is very interesting, showing that the infection is chiefly, if not always, got in the country; and further, that one village may have it while another has not, though, they somewhat closely resemble each other, as is the case with Gros Islet and Vieux Fort.

> *Dominica.* – Only 160 cases were examined, and of those 2 alone exhibited embryos of *filaria Demarquaii* [sic]; one a man from Batalie, a small village near the sea coast at the mouth of a valley, and the other a policeman who had lived all over the island; the latter had been a soldier in Sierra Leone in his

youth, but the former had never been out of the island. No cases were found in Roseau, the chief town of Dominica. This, again, points to a localised sphere of infection and, had time permitted the examination of further cases from Batalie, more from that area would probably have been found infected.

Barbadoes. – Filaria Demarquaii [sic] does not exist in this island 600 examinations from all parts of the island giving negative results, a fact already mentioned in a paper read at the [BMA] meeting at Cheltenham last summer [*see* above] on the malarial and filarial diseases of that island.

British Guiana. – Ozzard and Daniels have shown that the small sharp-tailed and blunt-tailed filariae of British Guiana are not got on the coast of that colony, but only in aboriginal Indians and others living in the interior, and the latter also pointed out that as many as 58.3 per cent. of those people were infected with one or other of those two parasites, the blunt-tailed predominating over the sharp-tailed.[4] In British Guiana 163 pure-blooded Indians were examined by me in different parts of the interior, and out of this number 105, or 64.4 per cent., a slightly higher figure than that of Daniels, were found to be infected with *filaria perstans* or *Demarquaii* [sic]. Double infections were found in 38, *perstans* alone in 56 instances, and *Demarquaii* [sic] alone in 11, giving 49 cases of the latter out of 163 Indians examined, or 30.01 per cent. This gives relatively a much higher percentage than St. Lucia and Dominica, but the general population of the whole island, including the towns, was considered in those cases, whereas in British Guiana only the specially-infected area was taken into account, the statistics of Georgetown and other parts of the coast cleared of bush which do not contain this parasite being omitted. The predominant physical feature for the occurrence of this parasite in British Guiana would seem to be the presence of forest and bush – that is, uncleared land. Georgetown and the cultivated strip of land along the coast is free, whereas on the Waini river, in the bush close to the sea, 9 out of 15 Waraw Indians living there were found to be infected. Conversely at Wismar, in the interior sixty miles up the Demerara river, where the forest has been cleared for a considerable extent to make room for a railway and other buildings in connection with a route to the gold fields, 25 people, Creoles and others, who had been living here for periods of two to ten years, on examination all gave negative results. As already stated by Daniels, negroes and others after living in appropriate parts of the interior are quite liable to infection, and this was confirmed by the fact of 3 out of 5 pure-blooded negroes who lived in the forest of the Pomeroon river being infected.

St Vincent. – The conditions and prevalence of the parasite here resemble that in St. Lucia, cases not being found in people living permanently in Kingstown, the chief town of the island, but only in some country villages and districts. In Calliaqua, a village situated on the coast on sandy soil, with swampy ground between it and the sea, scrubby bush and swamps at its sides, and a background of rising hills, 8 out of 30 people, or 26.6 per cent., were found to be infected.

But was there any evidence that *Filaria demarquayi* (or *Filaria perstans*) was associated with any pathological manifestations?

The presence of the parental and embryonic forms of the *filaria Demarquaii* [sic] seems to give rise to no pathological effects or clinical symptoms [a conclusion which was later confirmed], the diagnosis being made only by an examination of the blood. As the habitat of the parent is in the loose connective tissue of the peritoneum, with perhaps the exception of setting up some slight local inflammation on its death, it cannot do much harm, as it does not implicate important structures, as in the case of *filaria nocturna*. Through the kindness of the doctors in the Colonial hospital of Georgetown, Demerara, a necroscopy of an Indian, who had during life a few sharp-tailed embryos in his blood, was obtained: though a prolonged search of some hours was made the parental forms were not found.

It may be noted here in regard to the question of relationship between *filaria perstans* and sleeping sickness [an association favoured by Manson] that though the parasite, as has been shown above, abounds in the interior of British Guiana, no cases of this disease were seen and the Indians were unaware of its existence. Mr. Perkins, acting commissioner of gold mines, who has travelled extensively in the interior, informed me that he had never seen or heard of such cases amongst the Indians.[5]

David Grove (*see* Chapter 2) has summarised the history of research on *Filaria demarquayi* during and subsequent to Low's researches: In 1902, Low reported that he had compared microfilariae of *F. demarquayi* from St Lucia, Dominica and St Vincent with microfilariae of *M. ozzardi* from British Guiana, and concluded that they were identical. With recognition that *F. demarquayi* and *F. ozzardi* were synonymous, the correct name for the helminth appeared to be *Filaria demarquayi*, since Manson had first described this parasite in an 1897 paper. However, because this name had already been used for *W. bancrofti* by Zune,[6] Railliet proposed the designation *F. juncea*.[7] Leiper later pointed out that the second name given by Manson, *F. ozzardi*, had priority.[8] In 1914, Biglieri and Araoz discovered a microfilaria in individuals living in the province of Tucumán in northern Argentina, and named it *F. tucumani*;[9] this parasite was later shown, however, to be synonymous with the microfilaria of *F. ozzardi*.[10] In 1929, Faust instigated the genus *Mansonella* in honour of Manson, with this parasite as the prototype and sole species.[11] When Chaubaud and Bain reclassified the *Dipetalonema* group in 1976, they omitted *M. ozzardi* because they considered it insufficiently known for taxonomic consideration.[12] In 1982, Orihel and Eberhard redescribed the species and redefined the genus, using material obtained by infection of experimental monkeys (*Erythrocebus patas*).[13]

To Low's disappointment therefore, the host of *Filaria demarquayi* had still eluded him at the termination of his tour.

> On the analogy of the different species of filariae whose life-history have been completely worked out, namely, *filaria nocturna*,[14] *filaria immitis* and *filaria recondita*, *filaria Demarquaii* [sic] must also possess an intermediate host to allow of the further development and growth of the embryos and their reintroduction into man.
>
> While in St. Lucia I found by direct infection experiments on mosquitos reared from larvae, *Culex fatigans*, *Stegomyia fasciata* [= *A. aegypti*], *Culex taeniatus*, and *Anopheles albipes*, to be inefficient as intermediate hosts for this parasite and lately in British Guiana several other insects, mosquitos and others

were examined in an Indian settlement on the Pomeroon river in the interior of British Guiana with negative results, 71 per cent. of the inhabitants being infected with sharp or blunt-tailed parasites.

The blood-sucking insects were caught when they came to feed at night, as it was impossible to rear all those from larvae. The commonest night feeder there was a small chocolate brown mosquito with palps as long as its proboscis, not, however, resembling an *Anopheles*; it may represent a new genus altogether. Over 30 of these were dissected, but with the exception of a few dead embryos [microfilariae] in the semi-digested stomach blood of one, none were seen in any of the other tissues, thus showing them to be inefficient. A large yellow mosquito resembling an *aëdes* was another fairly common form, and it gave similar results to the former, in two instances dead and degenerated blunt and sharp-tailed embryos being seen in the stomach blood.

Many other mosquitos of the rarer genera frequented the huts and fed readily on the inmates; but though nothing was found in those dissected, yet the numbers were much too small positively to exclude them. Twelve fleas (*Pulex irritans*) and many chiggers (*Pulex penetrans*) from infected cases were examined but nothing was ever noted in them.

Though these observations were all negative some blood-sucking insect must nevertheless act as an intermediate host, and from the facts stated above, in reference to the sharply-defined country or forest areas in which persons infected by the parasite occur, it is very likely that it is an insect or insects with a similarly restricted distribution possibly only occurring at certain seasons of the year.[15]

Grove (*see* Chapter 2) has also provided an 'up-date' on the *host* of *F. demarquayi*. He reminded his readership that Low in 1901–02 attempted to determine the vector of the parasite by exposing infected patients to *Culex fatigans* (= *quinquefasciatus*), *Stegomyia fasciata* (= *Aëdes aegypti*), *C. taeniatus* and *Anopheles albipes*, but found that they were all refractory to infection. Subsequently, he caught and dissected a variety of blood-sucking insects (*see* above) feeding on inhabitants in a heavily endemic area of British Guiana, but again with negative results. In 1933, Buckley in St Vincent indicated that microfilariae of *M. ozzardi* were taken up by, and developed, in midges of the genus *Culicoides*,[16] especially *C. furens*.[17] Many years later, Nelson and Davies showed that *C. phlebotomus* was a vector in Trinidad,[18] while blackflies of the *Simulium* species, were implicated in transmission in parts of South America.[19]

Interestingly, there is still no evidence, as Manson had predicted, of any *pathological* consequences of an *M. ozzardi* infection. There now seems little doubt that the vast majority of infected individuals are symptomless; although articular pain, headache, fever and pruritis have variously been reported, their causative association with this nematode helminth has *not* been proved.

Yellow fever in St Lucia

At St Lucia, Low was confronted with the difficult problem of differentiating malignant malaria (*P falciparum* infection) from yellow fever (*see* Chapter 8). There was enormous difficulty in differentiating the two until Laveran's discovery of 1880 was widely accepted.[20] This led Low to summarise the *clinical* differences between the two, which cannot be bettered today:

> [The difficulty is especially relevant] as [William] Osler [1849–1919] states, in 'the early stages of an epidemic', and it is therefore exceedingly important that one should come to a definite conclusion quickly, first, to prevent the spread of the disease; and, secondly, to settle whether quarantine should or should not be imposed on the affected area.
>
> As regards the Lesser Antilles, where yellow fever is not endemic, this matter of diagnosis has in the past frequently proved a difficulty, some of the local physicians holding that in certain small epidemics real yellow fever has been present, whilst others maintain that it has not, the latter class explaining their position by the assumption that the cases were pernicious types of the malignant malaria so common in those islands. Clinically, there is no doubt that the two diseases may closely resemble each other; and though a combination of several well-marked features may encourage suspicion of yellow fever, not one of those features taken individually is sufficient for reliable diagnosis.

Briefly the common symptoms of the two diseases are as follows:

The Facial Appearance. – Much stress has been laid on the facial appearance in yellow fever, the flushing of the skin, the injection of the eyes, their ferrety appearance, and the anxious expression. Though those are well marked in certain cases, in others they are not so evident, and in cases of malarial fever flushing of the face and injection of the conjunctivae are by no means uncommon.

The Condition of the Tongue. – The same difficulty may be said to exist in regard to the tongue. It is true that pictures more or less characteristic of the appearance of this organ in the two diseases may be encountered – namely, the broad, flabby tongue of the one, and the sharp-pointed tongue of the other with its bright red edges and thickly-furred dorsum, but varying intermediate types are apt to confront one and to render it difficult to say which disease is present.

The Skin. – The skin may be hot and dry or moist in both diseases, depending on the time the cases are examined and on extraneous circumstances, such as temperature and clothing. Guitéras lays stress on the early appearance of jaundice in yellow fever, being recognizable in the conjunctiva, according to him, when carefully looked for, as early as the first morning. Sternberg, however, puts the oncoming of this feature as late as the third day, and the series of cases I have seen correspond to this. Osler [*see* above] notes the absence of early jaundice in malaria, stating 'that the colour of the skin is rarely changed within four or five days'; but then it must be remembered that the patient may have suffered from malaria before, and a fresh infection may show a certain amount of jaundice the relic of the previous attack. The general yellow colouring of the skin is not constant. In some cases of yellow fever it is entirely absent, though this is not the rule, whereas in some cases of malaria it is very marked. The same thing may be said of the different forms of petechiae which may be found in both diseases.

Temperature and Pulse. – The relation of the temperature to the pulse is one of importance in distinguishing the two diseases from each other, the gradual slowing of the latter, even when the temperature is still high, being specially indicative of yellow fever, *the rate often sinking as low as 40 beats per minute* [author's italics]. This, as far as my own experience goes, I have not seen in malaria.

Albuminuria. – Albuminuria, which has been considered so diagnostic of yellow fever, is exceedingly common in many of the severe types of malaria, and may be present in large amounts, a long series of cases examined in St. Lucia showing this very well. Osler [*see* above] states 'that it is rarely present in the urine so early as the second day in a malarial infection'.

Epigastric Pain. – This is common in yellow fever, especially on applying slight pressure in the region of the epigastrium, but this may easily be mistaken for the hepatic pain of the congested liver of malaria. Enlargement of the liver and spleen cannot be relied on for diagnosis, as they are not detectable in all forms of even the acutest malaria. When present they are suggestive of the latter disease.

Vomiting. – Bilious vomiting is an early feature in both diseases. Unfortunately, though rare, vomiting of black material may occur in what are known as the haemorrhagic forms of malarial fever, and on the other hand the black vomit so typical of yellow fever may never appear, this being especially so in the milder forms of the disease.

Haematuria. – This is got in both diseases as is also the case with melaena. Haemoglobinuria is got in blackwater fever – so far as is known a form of malaria; it does not occur in yellow fever.

Nervous System. – There is nothing positively characteristic in this system. The headache of yellow fever is more localized in the frontal and circumorbital regions, and is said to be more intense. Pains in the loins and limbs are frequent in both. Active delirium or coma may occur in either.

One must remember that there is no reason why a malarial subject should not develop yellow fever during an epidemic; the diagnosis in such a case would be a difficult one.[21]

He proceeded to outline the *laboratory* differences between the two infections:

… we possess an almost decisive method of at once determining between the two diseases – namely, *the examination of the blood for the malarial parasite* [author's italics]. It is true that in some cases the parasites of malignant malaria may be extremely scanty in the peripheral blood, and repeated search may be necessary to find them; but, as a rule, this does not hold good, one or two glances through the microscope often being sufficient to clear up the matter, parasites and corroborative evidence in the shape of pigmented leucocytes being seen. *Of course quinine must not have been administered before the examination of the blood is made; if this drug has been recently given a negative result is of no value* [author's italics].

The general and frequent use of quinine in malarious regions forms a real difficulty in the matter of diagnosis, because many people on the slightest indication of any fever at once dose themselves; one must always remember this in attempting a microscopic diagnosis.

Gray, of St. Lucia, has lately made differential counts of the leucocytes [*see* Chapter 8], and found in several cases of yellow fever that the large mononuclear leucocytes were normal, whereas in malaria, as Christophers[22] and Stephens,[23] and others have lately pointed out [wrote Low], their increase forms a diagnostic point of considerable importance. One case examined by myself substantiates this, but in a case examined by Guitéras [*see* above] over a period of several days they varied considerably, so that further research on this point is required. In Guitéras's case an enumeration of the red cells was also made and showed no diminution in the number of those elements.[24]

However, at *post mortem* Low considered diagnosis to be straightforward:

... presence of the characteristic malarial pigment, parasites localized in the brain, spleen, or gastric mucosa, at once tell us that the case is one of malaria; whereas in yellow fever these are absent and the liver shows the typical fatty degeneration.

In conclusion, therefore, one may state that it is of extreme importance to examine the blood carefully when called on to decide whether a case is one of pernicious malaria or yellow fever, and this especially so at the commencement of an epidemic when doubt may exist as to the nature of the disease.

Later on, when the epidemic is at its height, the rapid spread, the high death-rate, and the persistent occurrence of groups of symptoms in a large number of cases from the same areas will indicate clearly that yellow fever is present.[25]

Later references to the Caribbean expedition

Low continued referring to his Caribbean experience many years later. An overview, based on a paper read before the Society of Tropical Medicine and Hygiene in January 1908 was, for example, published in *The Lancet*. In this, he used three species of filaria: *nocturna, demarquayi*, and *perstans*, to illustrate problems in explaining the distribution of infective disease in the tropics.[26] Low also drew on his Caribbean experiences to argue *against* the likelihood of a reservoir of yellow fever in various species of sub-human primate.[27] (Sir) Andrew Balfour[28] had introduced this possibility in *The Lancet* for 1914.[29] Low was shortly to become interested, at Manson's direction, in *Filaria perstans*, and its possible role as the causative agent of *sleeping sickness*.[30] When writing about the geographical distribution of this helminth following his Ugandan expedition (*see* Chapter 1) he again referred to the Caribbean experience.

> *Filaria perstans*, as Daniels and Ozzard first pointed out, is very common amongst the aboriginal Indians in the interior of British Guiana, though not being found in Georgetown and the coast adjoining.
>
> While studying filarial disease in the West Indies in 1901 I did not once meet with it in the blood of large numbers of individuals examined in St. Kitts, Dominica, St. Lucia, Barbadoes, St. Vincent, Grenada, or Trinidad, but, as already mentioned, it was exceedingly common in British Guiana. Out of a total of 163 Indians seen in different parts of the dense tropical forests no fewer than 94, or 57.6 per cent., exhibited the parasite in their blood, 56 of those being pure infections, while in the other 38 it was associated with sharp-tailed embryos. Although it is not found in Georgetown and in New Amsterdam, nor the cultivated strip of the coast lying between in those two towns, it is common on the coast to the north near the Venezuelan boundary where the forests come down to the sea, Warau

Indians living at the mouth of the Waini river being found to be infected.

There is little doubt that the same parasite, if looked for, would be found in Dutch and French Guiana, Brazil, and in parts of Venezuela where the tropical forests are dense, and its distribution therefore is probably a much more extensive one in South America than we at present know of.[31]

Overall assessment of the Caribbean expedition

The degree of industry exhibited by Low during his Caribbean expedition is impressive. Although his observations and efforts at prevention of *P falciparum* infection, yellow fever, and the various filariases (most notably the lymphatic variety) probably had a limited long-term outcome, there is no doubt that taken in the context of the time, he made many important contributions to entomology, parasitology, and 'medicine in the tropics'.

A later account summarised Low's researches during tenure of his Scholarship:

> ... on the 26th December, 1900, ... Low left for the West Indies to investigate filarial and other tropical diseases. He visited St. Lucia, Dominica, Barbados, St. Vincent, St. Kitts, Grenada, Trinidad, and British Guiana. In addition to estimating the prevalence of filariasis in these different areas, experimental work on the life-history and other points in connection with these parasites were worked out. Later, at the request of the Governor of Barbados [Sir Frederic Hodgson], Low instituted sanitary courses and lectures on the destruction of mosquitos as a means of freeing the West Indian Islands from yellow fever, filariasis, and other diseases.
>
> A series of lectures of a similar nature were also delivered in St. Kitts. In December 1901, an outbreak of yellow fever having appeared in St. Lucia, ... Low returned to that island and cooperated with the army doctors in stamping out the disease. Further useful work on mosquito destruction by fumigating and destruction of breeding-places was conducted here.
>
> Low then proceeded to British Guiana, and visited many of the tribes of aboriginal Indians who inhabit the primeval

forest. Here a peculiar form of filariasis from which they suffer was investigated. After finishing this work ... Low returned to England in April 1902.[32]

References and Notes

1 St G Gray, G C Low. Malarial fever in St. Lucia, W.I. *Br med J* 1902; i: 193–4.

2 G C Low. The absence of *Anopheles* in Barbadoes, W.I. *Br med J* 1902; i: 200.

3 G C Low. Malarial and filarial disease in Barbadoes, West Indies. *Br med J* 1902; i: 1472–3.

4 A T Ozzard, C W Daniels. A supposed new species of filaria sanguinis hominis found in the interior of British Guiana. *Br Guiana Med Ann* 1897; 9: 24–7.

5 G C Low. Notes on *Filaria Demarquayii*. *Br med J* 1902; i: 196–7.

6 A Zune. *Urine chylenses et hématochyleuses*. Paris 1891: 82.

7 A Railliet. *Précis de parasitologie humaine. Maladies parasitaires dues à des végé-taux et à des animaux*. M Neveu-Lemaire (ed). Paris: J Lamarre 1908: 712. (Quoted by D I Grove, see Note 13.)

8 R T Leiper. Observations on certain helminths of man. *Trans Soc trop Med Hyg* 1913; 6: 265–97.

9 R Biblieri, J L Araoz. '*Contribución al estudio de una nueva filariosis humana encontrada en la República Argentina (Tucumán) ocasionada por la "Filaria tucumana".*' *Primera conferencia de la Sociedad Sud-Americana de Higiene, Microbiologio y Patologia*, Buenos Aires, 17–24 Septiembre, 1916. Buenos Aires, 1917. (Quoted by D I Grove.)

10 H Vogel. *Ueber Mikrofilaria demarquayi und die Mikrofilaria aus Tucuman in Argentinien Abhundinngen aus dem Gebiet des Auslandkunde*. Hamburg Universität 1927; 26: 573–8. (Quoted by D I Grove.)

11 E C Faust. *Human helminthology. A manual for clinicians, sanitarians and medical zoologists*. Philadelphia: Lea & Febiger 1929: 616.

12 A G Chabaud, O Bain. *La lignée Dipetalonema. Nouvel essai de classification. Archives de Parasitologie Humaine et Comparée*. 1976; 51: 365–7.

13 T C Orihel, M L Eberhard. *Mansonella ozzardi*: a redescription with comments on its taxonomic relationships. *Am J trop Med Hyg* 1982; 31: 1142–7; D I Grove. *A History of Human Helminthology*. Wallingford, Oxon: CAB International 1990: 734–6.

14 G C Low. The development of *filaria nocturna* in different species of mosquitos. *Br med J* 1901; i: 1336–7.

15 *Op cit*. See Note 5 above.

16 J J C Buckley. Some observations on two West Indian parasites of man. *Proc R Soc Med (Section of Comparative Medicine)* 1933; 27: 134–5.

17 J J C Buckley. On the development, in *Culicoides furens* Poey, of *Filaria* (= *Mansonella*) *ozzardi* Manson, 1897. *J Helminth* 1934; 12: 99–118.

18 G S Nelson, J B Davies. Observations on *Mansonella ozzardi* in Trinidad. *Trans R Soc trop Med Hyg* 1970; 70: 16–17.

19 U Undiano. *Importancia y actualización del nuevo concepta de la patogenicidad de la mansoneliasis. Rev Facul Ciencias Médicas de la Universidad Nacional de Cordoba.* 1966; 24: 183–9; M A Tidwell, M Tidwell, P Muñoz de Hoyos. Development of *Mansonella ozzardi* in a black fly species of the *Simulium Sanguineum* groups from eastern Vaupes, Columbia. *Am J trop Med Hyg* 1980; 29: 1209–14. [*See also*: *Op cit*. See Note 13 above (Grove).]

20 C Lloyd, J L S Coulter. *Medicine and the Navy 1200–1900*. 4 (1815–1900). London: E & S Livingstone Ltd 1963: 173–96.

21 G C Low. The differential diagnosis of yellow fever and malignant malaria. *Br med J* 1902; ii: 860–1.

22 **Sir (Samuel) Rickard Christophers** FRS (1873–1978) was a leading protozoologist and specialist in Tropical Medicine. He was educated at University College, Liverpool, and proceeded to South America and India (where he served in the research branch of the Indian Medical Service). He was subsequently Professor of Malarial Studies at the London School of Hygiene and Tropical Medicine. [*See also*: Anonymous. Christophers, Brevet Col Sir (Samuel) Rickard. *Who Was Who, 1971–1980*. London: A & C Black 1981: 148–9; C Garnham. Christophers, Sir (Samuel) Rickard (1873–1978). In: H C G Matthew, B Harrison (eds). *Oxford Dictionary of National Biography*. Oxford: Oxford University Press 2004; 11: 559–60.]

23 **John William Watson Stephens** FRS (1865–1946) was an eminent parasitologist and tropical diseases expert. He received his training at Gonville and Caius College, Cambridge, and St Bartholomew's Hospital, London. After service in India and British Central Africa, Stephens spent most of his career at the Liverpool School of Tropical Medicine, where he became Walter Myers Professor of Tropical Medicine. [*See also*: Anonymous. Stephens, John William Watson. *Who Was Who, 1941–1950*. 5th ed. London: A & C Black 1980: 1099; W F Bynum. Stephens, John William Watson (1865–1946). In: H C G Matthew, B Harrison (eds). *Oxford Dictionary of National Biography*. Oxford: Oxford University Press 2004; 52: 476–7.]

24 *Op cit*. See Note 21 above.

25 *Ibid*.

26 G C Low. The unequal distribution of filariasis in the tropics. *Lancet* 1908; i: 279–81. G C Low. The unequal distribution of filariasis in the tropics. *Trans Soc trop Med Hyg*. 1908; 1: 84–96.

27 G C Low. Monkeys as reservoirs for the virus of yellow fever. *Lancet* 1914; i: 1357–8.

28 **Sir Andrew Balfour FRCP** (1873–1931). Anonymous. *Times Lond* 1931: 2 February; C M Wenyon. Sir Andrew Balfour. *Nature, Lond* 1931, 127: 279–81; Anonymous. Sir Andrew Balfour. *Lancet* 1931 i: 325–7; P H Manson-Bahr. Sir Andrew Balfour. *Br med J* 1931; i 245–6; C M Wenyon. Sir Andrew Balfour. *Trans R Soc trop Med Hyg* 1931, 24: 655–9; Anonymous. *Munk's Roll*. 5. London Royal College of Physicians: 19–29; P Manson-Bahr. *History of the School of*

Tropical Medicine in London (1899–1949). London 1956: H K Lewis, 167–73, 216–18; Anonymous. Balfour, Sir Andrew. *Who Was Who, 1929–1940.* 2nd ed. London A & C Black 1967: 57; A S Macnalty, M E Gibson. Balfour, Sir Andrew (1873–1931). In: H C G Matthew, B Harrison (eds). *Oxford Dictionary of National Biography.* Oxford: Oxford University Press 2004; 3: 493–4.

29 A Balfour. The wild monkey as a reservoir for the virus of yellow fever. *Lancet* 1914; i: 1176–8. [*See also*: G C Cook. *Tropical Medicine: an illustrated history of the pioneers.* London: Academic Press 2007: 227.]

30 G C Cook. Correspondence from Dr George Carmichael Low to Dr Patrick Manson during the first Ugandan sleeping sickness expedition. *J med Biog* 1993; 1: 215–29.

31 G C Low. Filaria perstans. *Br med J* 1903; i: 722–4; G C Low. Filaria perstans. *J trop Med Hyg* 1903; 6: 180–2, 198–9.

32 Seamen's Hospital Society; The London School of Tropical Medicine. '*A short account of "The Craggs Prize", from 1899 to 1911.*' Presented at a meeting at the Mansion House, presided over by the Rt Hon The Lord Mayor, Wednesday 28th February 1912: 4.

Epilogue

In 1901–02 Patrick Manson (then in his mid-fifties) was at the height of his administrative powers; however, his seminal clinical investigation which demonstrated the man-mosquito component of the lymphatic filaria life-cycle had been carried out over two decades previously – in the 1870s. Clearly, he was the dominant figure (apart perhaps from Joseph Chamberlain [1836–1914])[1] – Secretary of State for the Colonies – at the newly founded London School of Tropical Medicine (LSTM) and his thoughts and actions must have exerted a profound influence on his 'disciples'.

Obviously, it must have been a great privilege to be elected to the staff of the LSTM at that time. However, there were significant disadvantages: Manson claimed that a host of diseases resulted from a filaria infection; he felt for example (erroneously) that the 'negro lethargy' of Uganda was a result of *Filaria (Mansonella) perstans* infection. Whether he directly influenced Low in his pursuit for the intermediate host of *F demarquayi* remains unknown; however, the 'climate' at the LSTM must have been such that embarkation on such a project was potentially worthwhile. Low largely failed therefore in two major quests: this Caribbean enter-prise *and* the first Royal Society expedition to Uganda.[2] Both of these researches were carried out when Low's research capabilities would have been maximal (i.e. when he was around 30 years old).

However, on the positive side, Low did much to delineate the disease spectrum at various Windward Islands. He also conveyed the important 'message' that *preventive* strategies (at that time *not* widely appreciated) should be implemented, in order to limit the mosquito population and hence the elimination of malaria, elephantiasis and yellow fever; he thus contributed significantly to disease *prevention* in the Caribbean – a major undertaking of the Liverpool School in West Africa.

As a 'bonus', while on this expedition, Low encountered a yellow fever outbreak; his dealing with this (he had engaged no previous experience of handling such an event) was exemplary.

Low was obviously fascinated by the geographical diversity in the distribution of various species, including insects, parasites and above all human disease. Much of his work in the West Indies was therefore not too dissimilar from that of Charles Darwin (1809–82), carried out in the Galapagos Islands.[3]

The fact that he remains such an underrated pioneer of the formal discipline of *tropical (colonial) medicine* must rest to some extent therefore on Manson's shoulders.

References and Notes

1   P T Marsh. Chamberlain, Joseph (Joe) (1836–1914). In: H C G Matthew, B Harrison (eds). *Oxford Dictionary of National Biography.* Oxford: Oxford University Press 2004; 10: 923–34.

2   G C Cook. *Tropical Medicine: an illustrated history of the pioneers.* London: Academic Press 2007: 133–5. [*See also*: G C Cook. Correspondence from Dr George Carmichael Low to Dr Patrick Manson during the first Ugandan sleeping sickness expedition. *J med Biog* 1993; 1: 215–29.]

3   A Desmond, J Moore. *Darwin.* London: Michael Joseph 1991: 808. [*See also*: P Davies. The 'coffin brig' that sailed the ultimate voyage of discovery. *Times, Lond* 2009; 12 February: S4–S5.]

Appendices

Appendix I

Letter written by Samuel Miller Low to Dr Patrick Manson.

Letter XXVII

ASHLEA
MONIFIETH N8
19th January 1902

Dear Sir,

The enclosed correspondence has been kindly handed to me by Mr. F Sharp for perusal & I now return it to you as requested with many thanks. It gives me great pleasure to know that my son continues to merit your good opinion & I can assure you his mother & I duly appreciate the many kindnesses he has from first to last received from you.

    With kind regards and believe me,

Yours faithfully
Sam. M. Low.

Dr. Patrick Manson C.M.G.
London

Appendix II

Low's major contributions to medical/scientific literature*

(publications relevant to the Caribbean expedition are shown in bold font)

1900:
1 A recent observation on Filaria nocturna in Culex: probable mode of infection of man. *Br med J* 1900; i: 1456–7.
2 [*with* L W Sambon.] On the resting position of Anopheles. *Br med J* 1900; ii: 1158.

1902:
3 **[*with* St G Gray.] Malarial fever in St. Lucia, W.I. *Br med J* 1902; i: 193–4.**
4 **Notes on Filaria demarquaii. *Br med J* 1902; i: 196–7.**
5 **The absence of *Anopheles* in Barbadoes, W.I. *Br med J* 1902; i: 200.**
6 **Malarial and filarial diseases in Barbadoes, West Indies. *Br med J* 1902; i: 1472–3.**
7 **The differential diagnosis of yellow fever and malignant malaria. *Br med J* 1902; ii: 860–1.**
8 Filariasis in St Kitts, WI. *J trop Med* 1902; 5: 117–9.
9 G C Low. Filarial lymphangitis. *Br Guiana Med Ann* 1902; 14: 1–9. [*See also*: *J trop Med* 1902; 5: 255–6].

1903:
10 **Filaria perstans. *Br med J* 1903; i: 722–4.**
11 [*with* C Christy, A Castellani.] The etiology, pathology, and symptoms of sleeping sickness. *Br med J* 1903; ii: 1427–9.
12 **Filaria perstans. *J trop Med* 1903; 6: 180–2, 198–9.**
13 [*with* A Castellani.] Climatic bubo in Uganda. *J trop Med* 1903; 6: 379–80.
14 *Filaria perstans* and its relationship to sleeping sickness. Reports of the Sleeping Sickness Commission. Royal Society: Harrison & Sons 1903; no II: 64–9.

---

* It should be noted that several of Low's publications appeared in both *J trop Med* or *Trans Soc trop Med Hyg* and also *Br med J*.

1904:
15 [*with* P Manson.] The Leishman-Donovan body and tropical splenomegaly. *Br med J* 1904; i: 183–6.
16 [*with* F W Mott.] The examination of the tissues of the case of sleeping sickness in a European. *Br med J* 1904; i: 1000–2.
17 [*with* P Manson.] The Leishman-Donovan body. *Br med J* 1904; i: 1251.
18 [*with* P Manson.] The Leishman-Donovan body in ulcerated surfaces; a possible route of its escape from the human body. *Br med J* 1904; ii: 11.
19 A new filaria in a monkey. *J trop Med* 1904; 7: 2–3.
20 Filaria perstans and the suggestion that it belongs to the genus Tylenchus (Bastian). *Lancet* 1904; i: 420–1.
21 'Filaria perstans'. *Lancet* 1904; i: 752–3.

1905:
22 A note on filaria gigas. *Br med J* 1905; i: 1329–30.
23 As filarias. *Med mod Porto* 1905; 12: 297–300.

1907:
24 Sleeping sickness. In: C Allbutt (ed.). *System of Medicine* 8th ed. London 1907; ii (part 2): 208–26.

1908:
25 Sleeping sickness. *Hospital* 1908; 43: 359–62.
26 **Filariasis. *Hospital* 1908; 44: 123**.
27 **The unequal distribution of filariasis in the tropics. *Lancet* 1908; i: 279–81.**
28 **The unequal distribution of filariasis in the tropics. *Trans Soc trop Med Hyg* 1908; I: 84–96, 105–8.**

1909:
29 Filaria philippinensis. *J trop Med Hyg* 1909; 12: 256.
30 A case of Malta fever from northern Nigeria. *Trans Soc trop Med Hyg* 1909; 2: 202–5.

1910:
31 Tropical haematology: Romanowski's chromatin stain and its modifications. *Hospital* 1910; 47: 485–6.
32 Insects as carriers of tropical diseases. *Hospital* 1910; 49: 281–4.
33 The transmission in nature of *Trypanosoma gambiense*. *J trop Med Hyg* 1910; 13: 209.

1911:
34 Filaria loa. *J trop Med Hyg* 1911; 14: 5–8.
35 The etiology of elephantiasis. *J trop Med Hyg* 1911; 14: 83–6.

1912:

36 The absence of eosinophilia in chronic cases of helminthiasis. *J State Med* 1912; 20: 413–7.

37 Persistence of eosinophilia and persistence or absence of embryos in peripheral blood in a case of *Filaria loa* infection. *J trop Med Hyg* 1912; 15: 38–9.

38 The life of filarial embryos outside the body. *J trop Med Hyg* 1912; 15: 338–9.

39 [*with* P Bahr.] A case of tuberculosis with special involvement of the heart. *Lancet* 1912; i: 362–3.

40 The development of *Filaria immitis* in the mosquito. *Trans Soc trop Med Hyg* 1912; 5: 226.

1913:

41 The administration of emetine by the mouth in amoebic dysentery. *Br med J* 1913; i: 1369–70.

42 Discussion on filariasis. *Br med J* 1913; ii: 1298–1302.

43 [*with* A Castellani.] The *rôle* played by fungi in sprue. *J trop Med Hyg* 1913; 16: 33–5.

44 Filaria loa cases: continuation reports. *J trop Med Hyg* 1913; 16: 118–20.

45 [*with* C M Wenyon.] Cell inclusions in the leucocytes of blackwater fever and other tropical diseases. *J trop Med Hyg* 1913; 16: 161–3.

1914:

46 **Yellow fever. *Br med J* 1914; ii: 1120.**

47 Arthritis in sprue. *J trop Med Hyg* 1914; 17: 1–2.

48 [*with* C M Wenyon.] The occurrence of certain structures in the erythrocytes of guinea-pigs and their relationship to the so-called parasite of yellow fever. *J trop Med Hyg* 1914; 17: 369–72.

49 **Monkeys as reservoirs for the virus of yellow fever. *Lancet* 1914; i: 1357–8.**

50 Recent researches on emetine and its value as a therapeutic agent in amoebiasis and other diseases. *Proc R Soc Med* (Therap & Parmacol Sect) 1914; 7: 41–9.

1915:

51 The treatment of epidemic cerebrospinal meningitis. *Br med J* 1915; i: 376.

52 The treatment of amoebic dysentery. *Br med J* 1915; ii: 714–6.

53 [*with* C M Wenyon.] The so-called parasite of yellow fever. *J trop Med Hyg* 1915; 18: 55–6.

54 A case of oriental sore treated by antimonium tartaratum (tartar emetic) locally. *J trop Med Hyg* 1915; 18: 258–60.

1916:

55 The treatment of lamblia infections. *Br med J* 1916; i: 450.

56 [*with* H B Newham.] A case of ulcerating granuloma successfully treated by intravenous injection of antimony. *Br med J* 1916; ii: 387–9.

57 A case of amoebic abscess of the liver occurring twenty years after the original attack of dysentery. *Br med J* 1916; ii: 867–8.

58 Two chronic amoebic dysentery carriers treated by emetine, with some remarks on the treatment of lamblia, blastocystis, and *B. coli* infectons. *J trop Med Hyg* 1916; 19: 29–34.

59 [*with* C Dobell.] Three cases of entamoeba histolytica infection treated with emetine bismuth iodide. *Lancet* 1916; ii: 319–21.

60 [*with* C Dobell.] A note on the treatment of lamblia infections. *Lancet* 1916; ii: 1053–4.

61 Amoebic dysentery. *Practitioner* 1916; 96: 320–31.

62 Dysenteries other than amoebic. *Practitioner* 1916; 96: 510–25.

63 An interesting case of eosinophilia. *Trans Soc trop Med Hyg* 1916; 9: 77–81.

64 An interesting case of syphilitic pyrexia in an Indian native. The value of a positive Wassermann reaction in diagnosis. *Trans Soc trop Med Hyg* 1916; 9: 235–41.

1917:

65 [*with* H B Newham.] Intravenous injections of antimony in the treatment of malaria. *Br med J* 1917; i: 295.

66 Emetine diarrhoea. *Br med J* 1917; ii: 484.

67 Further experiences with emetine bismuth iodide in amoebic dysentery, amoebic hepatitis, and general amoebiasis. *Lancet* 1917; i: 482–5.

68 The 'haemogregarine' of trench fever. *Lancet* 1917; ii: 473.

69 The history of the use of intravenous injections of tartar emetic (*Antimonium Tartaratum*) in tropical medicine. *Trans Soc trop Med Hyg* 1917; 10: 37–42.

70 Diemenal in the treatment of malarial fever. *Trans Soc trop Med Hyg* 1917; 10: 97–9.

71 [*with* H B Newham.] A case of ulcerating granuloma refractory to intravenous injections of antimony, X-rays and other forms of treatment. *Trans Soc trop Med Hyg* 1917; 10: 109–13.

1918:

72 Emetine bismuth iodide in the treatment of amoebic dysentery. *Br med J* 1918; i: 188.

73 [*with* R P Cockin.] A case of rat-bite fever treated successfully by injections of novarsenobillon. *Br med J* 1918; i: 203–4.

74 The life-history of Ascaris lumbricoides. *Br med J* 1918; i: 286.

75 A series of acute and subacute amoebic dysentery cases treated by emetine bismuth iodide and other drugs. *Trans Soc trop Med Hyg* 1918; 11: 155–67.

1919:

76 Antimony in the treatment of American leishmaniasis of the skin. *Br med J* 1919; i: 479–80.

77 Intravenous injections of antimonium tartaratum in kala-azar. *Br med J* 1919; i: 702–4.

78 Kala-azar in Mesopotamia and its incubation period. *Br med J* 1919; ii: 758–9.

79 A case of bilharzial disease treated by intravenous injections of antimonium tartaratum. *J trop Med Hyg* 1919; 22: 93–4.

80 [*with* H B G Newham.] A series of cases of bilharziasis treated by intravenous injections of antimonium tartaratum. *Lancet* 1919; ii: 633–6.

1920:

81 Some unusual forms of dysentery. *Br med J* 1920; i: 255–6.

82 [*with* P Manson-Bahr.] Filaria bancrofti in the production of elephantiasis and kindred diseases. *Br med J* 1920; ii: 233–5.

83 The treatment of bilharzial disease by antimonium tartaratum. *J State Med* 1920; 28: 283–9.

84 Case of oriental sore cured by intravenous injections and innuctions of antimonium tartaratum. *J State Med* 1920; 28: 354–5.

85 [*with* A L Gregg.] The uselessness of antimony in the treatment of filariasis. *Lancet* 1920; ii: 551–2.

86 Filariasis. In: *Nelson Loose-Leaf Med.* Lond & NY 1920; ii: 464–9.

1921:

87 [*with* E J O'Driscoll.] A case of dibothriocephalus latus infection. *Br med J* 1921; i: 118.

88 [*with* E J O'Driscoll.] Further researches upon antimony in the treatment of filariasis. *Lancet* 1921; i: 221–2.

89 [*with* E J O'Driscoll.] Observations upon a case of filaria (loa) loa infection. *Lancet* 1921; i: 798–800.

1922:

90 [*with* H B G Newham.] Case of trypanosomiasis from Portuguese East Africa apparently cured. *Br med J* 1922; i: 96–7.

91 [*with* P Manson-Bahr.] Preliminary note on the therapeutic action of Bayer '205' in nine cases of human trypanosomiasis. *Lancet* 1922; ii: 1265–7.

1923:

92 [*with* P Manson-Bahr.] The new trypanocidal remedies. 'Bayer 205'. *Br med J* 1923; i: 149.

93 [*with* P Manson-Bahr, J J Pratt, A L Gregg.] The treatment of liver abscess by aspiration, with an account of fifteen cases. *Lancet* 1923; i: 941–5.

94 [*with* P Manson-Bahr.] The treatment of human trypanosomiasis by 'Bayer 205'. *Trans R Soc trop Med Hyg* 1923; 16: 339–83.

95 Elephantiasis nostras; description of a case, with autopsy findings. *Trans R Soc trop Med Hyg* 1923; 17: 77–81.

96 [*with* C W Daniels.] Yaws; tropical sore; leprosy; madura foot; granuloma of the pudenda. In: C C Choyce (ed). *Choyce's System of Surgery* 1923; i: 887–903.

1924:

97 A case of rat-bite fever in England. *Recovery of the spirochaete from the blood.* *Br med J* 1924; i: 236.

98 The modern treatment of human trypanosomiasis. *J State Med* 1924; 32: 535–8.

99 Unusual varieties of Calabar swellings. With a note upon the aetiology of the condition. *Lancet* 1924; i: 594–5.

100 [*with* W E Cooke.] Bayer 'G. 1919' in the treatment of filariasis. *Lancet* 1924; ii: 903–4.

101 [*with* J T Duncan.] The etiology of blackwater fever. *Trans R Soc trop Med Hyg* 1924; 17: 201–4.

102 A second series of cases of human trypanosomiasis treated by 'Bayer 205': with an account of the after-histories of some of the first series. *Trans R Soc trop Med Hyg* 1924; 17: 464–73.

1925:

103 Recent observations upon the human Filariidae. *J State Med* 1925; 33: 415–8.

104 [*with* A L Gregg.] 'Smalarina' in malaria. *Lancet* 1925; i: 1339–41.

105 [*with* A L Gregg.] 'Smalarina' in malaria. *Trans R Soc trop Med Hyg* 1925; 19: 107.

1926:

106 [*with* J M H MacLeod, P Manson-Bahr, J H Sequeira.] Leprosy: its transmission and treatment. *Br med J* 1926; ii: 1141.

107 [*with* W E Cooke.] Climatic bubo and its treatment by 'protein shock' and aspiration. *J State Med* 1926; 34: 450–63.

108 [*with* W E Cooke.] A congenital case of kala-azar. *Lancet* 1926; ii: 1209–11.

109 Tropical Medicine. In: F W Price (ed). *A Textbook of the Practice of Medicine.* 2nd ed. London: Oxford University Press 1926: 318–44.

1927:

110 A series of kala-azar cases treated by antimony derivatives. *J State Med* 1927; 35: 591–4.

111 [*with* E G Sayers.] Early diagnosis of kala-azar. *J trop Med Hyg* 1927; 30: 46–8.

112 [*with* D Benton.] Sprue in natives. *J trop Med Hyg* 1927; 30: 193.

113 [*with* W E Cooke.] Blood transfusion in sprue. *Lancet* 1927; ii: 960–1.

114 Loa loa infection in central equatorial Africa. *Trans R Soc trop Med Hyg* 1927; 20: 514–5.

1928:

115 [*with* W E Cooke, P H Martin.] Blood transfusion in blackwater fever. *Lancet* 1928; ii: 645–7.

116 Sprue: an analytical study of 150 cases. *Quart J Med* 1928; 21: 523–34.

117 The history of the foundation of the Society of Tropical Medicine and Hygiene. *Trans R Soc trop Med Hyg* 1928; 22: 197–202.

1929:

118 Dysentery. *Livingstonian.* H E Jump (ed). London: Longmans, Green & Co 1929: 12–14.

119 A retrospect of tropical medicine from 1894 to 1914. *Trans R Soc trop Med Hyg* 1929; 23: 213–32.

120 An interesting case of kala-azar from the point of view of diagnosis. *Trans R Soc trop Med Hyg* 1929; 23: 305–8.

1930:

121 Non-specific protein therapy in elephantiasis. *Br med J* 1930; ii: 1065.

122 Climatic bubo: its diagnosis and treatment. *J R Nav Med Serv* 1930; 16: 272–5.

123 Climatic bubo: its diagnosis and treatment. *J State Med* 1930; 38: 638–40.

124 [*with* D S Dixon.] Elephantiasis treated by protein shock. *Lancet* 1930; i: 72–3.

125 [*with* D S Dixon.] Pseudo-sprue. *Trans R Soc trop Med Hyg* 1930; 23: 525–8.

126 Tropical myositis. *Trans R Soc trop Med Hyg.* 1930; 23: 547–8.

1931:

127 [*with* N H Fairley.] Observations on laboratory and hospital infections with yellow fever in England. *Br med J* 1931; i: 125–8.

128 Sir William John Richie Simpson CMG, MD, FRCP. *Br med J* 1931; ii: 633.

129 Some points in the pathology of filariasis: *Filaria bancrofti, Loa loa* and *Onchocerca volvulus* infections. *J State Med* 1931; 39: 594–8.

130 [*with* A B Cook.] Thrombo-phlebitis migrans: a report of two cases in Asiatics. *Lancet* 1931; i: 584–5.

131 Sir Andrew Balfour. *Trans R Soc trop Med Hyg* 1931; 24: 575–6.

1932:

132 Sir Ronald Ross. *Br med J* 1932; ii: 611.

133 [*with* R H Franklin.] New antimony preparations in the treatment of Mediterranean leishmaniasis and Japanese (or eastern) schistosomiasis. *Lancet* 1932; i: 395–6.

1933:

134 [*with* P H Manson-Bahr, A H Walters.] Some recent observations on filarial periodicity. With a clinical and laboratory report. *Lancet* 1933; i: 466–8.

135 The treatment of tropical intestinal diseases. *Practitioner* 1933; 131: 136–45.

136 Professor William Sydney Thayer MD, LLD. *Trans R Soc trop Med Hyg* 1933; 26: 404.

1934:

137 [*with* N H Fairley.] Fatal perforation of caecum in a case of sprue. *Br med J* 1934; ii: 678–9.

138 The skin conditions found in *Loa loa* infections. *J trop Med Hyg* 1934; 37: 359–60.

139 [*with* P H Manson-Bahr, A H Walters.] Further observations on filarial periodicity. With a laboratory report. *Lancet* 1934; ii: 531–5.

1935:
140 Tropical medicine; introductory address. *Br med J* 1935; ii: 715–7.
141 [*with* G R M Cordiner.] Case of *porocephalus* infection in a West African negro. *Trans R Soc trop Med Hyg* 1935; 28: 535–7.

1937:
142 Brief summary of development of tropical medicine. *Nocht Festschr* 1937: 271–2.
143 [*with* N H Fairley.] Tropical Medicine. In: *A Textbook of the Practice of Medicine.* 5th ed. London: Oxford University Press 1937: 191–234.

1941:
144 The nomenclature of the Pacific Filaria. *Trans R Soc trop Med Hyg* 1941; 35: 197–8.

1945:
145 Tribute to Manson's life and work. *Trans R Soc trop Med Hyg* 1945; 38: 417–20.

Minor contributions to the medical/scientific literature: discussions, demonstrations, etc

1907:
 1 Sleeping sickness. *Trans Soc trop Med Hyg* 1907; 1: 42.
 2 Oriental sore. *Trans Soc trop Med Hyg* 1907; 1: 48.

1908:
 3 Kala-azar. *Trans Soc trop Med Hyg* 1908; 1: 134–7.
 4 Pernicious malaria. *Trans Soc trop Med Hyg* 1908; 1: 148.
 5 Tropical lands and white races. *Trans Soc trop Med Hyg* 1908; 1: 217–20.
 6 African tick fever. *Trans Soc trop Med Hyg* 1908; 1: 263–4.
 7 Cerebrospinal fever in the Gold Coast. *Trans Soc trop Med Hyg* 1908; 2: 35–7.
 8 Plague in Bombay. *Trans Soc trop Med Hyg* 1908; 2: 110.
 9 Barbados. *Trans Soc trop Med Hyg* 1908; 2: 153.
10 The United States Board in the Philippines. *Trans Soc trop Med Hyg* 1908; 2: 194–7.

1909:
11 Beri-beri. *Trans Soc trop Med Hyg* 1909; 2: 239–40.
12 Recent advances in sleeping sickness. *Trans Soc trop Med Hyg* 1909; 3: 32–4.

13 The mechanism of infection in tick fever, and on the hereditary transmission of Spirochaeta Duttoni in the tick. *Trans Soc trop Med Hyg* 1909; 3: 97–8.

1910:
14 The nature and origin of Calabar swellings. *Trans Soc trop Med Hyg* 1910; 3: 251–3.
15 Recent advances in sleeping sickness. *Trans Soc trop Med Hyg* 1910; 4: 29.

1911:
16 The distribution and prevalence of yellow fever in West Africa. *Trans Soc trop Med Hyg* 1911; 4: 125–6.
17 Alastrim, amaas, or milk-pox. *Trans Soc trop Med Hyg* 1911; 4: 232.

1912:
18 Filariasis in Fiji. *Trans Soc trop Med Hyg* 1912; 5: 152–3.
19 The prophylaxis of trypanosomiasis in Nyasaland. *Trans Soc trop Med Hyg* 1912; 5: 327–8.

1913:
20 Recent advances in sleeping sickness. *Trans Soc trop Med Hyg* 1913; 6: 130.
21 The culture of malarial parasites and *Piroplasma canis*. *Trans Soc trop Med Hyg* 1913; 6: 229.
22 Mosquito reduction and the consequent eradication of malaria. *Trans Soc trop Med Hyg* 1913; 7: 74–6.

1914:
23 Researches on sprue. *Trans Soc trop Med Hyg* 1914; 7: 185–7.
24 An entoplasma. *Trans Soc trop Med Hyg* 1914; 7: 216, 218.
25 African trypanosomes pathogenic to man and animals. *Trans Soc trop Med Hyg* 1914; 8: 35, 36–7.

1915:
26 Bacillary dysentery. *Trans Soc trop Med Hyg* 1915; 8: 130, 134, 135, 136.
27 Epidemic of African tick fever among the troops in British Somaliland. *Trans Soc trop Med Hyg* 1915; 8: 208.
28 The etiology of *Leishmaniasis Americana*. *Trans Soc trop Med Hyg* 1915; 8: 229.

1916:
29 Intestinal parasites in northern Siam. *Trans Soc trop Med Hyg* 1916; 9: 92, 93.
30 The etiology of typhus. *Trans Soc trop Med Hyg* 1916; 9: 115–6.

1917:
31 The vomiting sickness of Jamaica. *Trans Soc trop Med Hyg* 1917; 10: 63.

32 Spontaneous disappearance of yellow fever from failure of the human host. *Trans Soc trop Med Hyg* 1917; 10: 132, 133–5, 135–6.

33 The distribution among foodstuffs of the substances required for the prevention of beriberi and scurvy. *Trans Soc trop Med Hyg* 1917; 10: 184–5, 186.

1918:

34 The geographical distribution of human diseases and their control. *Trans Soc trop Med Hyg* 1918; 11: 124.

35 A series of sixteen cases of blackwater fever occurring in the Eastern Mediterranean. *Trans Soc trop Med Hyg* 1918; 11: 151–3.

36 The presence of *Entamoeba histolytica* and *E coli* cysts in people who have not been out of England. *Trans Soc trop Med Hyg* 1918; 11: 295.

1920:

37 Trypanosomiasis. *Trans R Soc trop Med Hyg* 1920; 14: 47.

38 Relapsing fever. *Trans R Soc trop Med Hyg* 1920; 14: 106–7.

39 Filariasis. *Trans R Soc trop Med Hyg* 1920; 14: 109.

1921:

40 Trypanosomiasis. *Trans R Soc trop Med Hyg* 1921; 15: 28–31.

1922:

41 Researches in the western Pacific. *Trans R Soc trop Med Hyg* 1922; 16: 54.

42 Sprue. *Trans R Soc trop Med Hyg* 1922; 16: 132.

1923:

43 Tryparsamide in sleeping sickness. *Trans R Soc trop Med Hyg* 1923; 16: 416–7.

44 Emetine preparations for rectal and oral use. *Trans R Soc trop Med Hyg* 1923; 17: 33–5.

45 Yaws in Kenya Colony. *Trans R Soc trop Med Hyg* 1923; 17: 285.

1924:

46 The action of 'Bayer 205' in trypanosomiasis. *Trans R Soc trop Med Hyg* 1924; 17: 456–7.

47 Malaria during treatment of general paralysis. *Trans R Soc trop Med Hyg* 1924; 18: 36.

1926:

48 Chemotherapy of surra of horses and cattle. *Trans R Soc trop Med Hyg* 1926; 20: 71.

49 Chemotherapy and immunity reactions of schistosomiasis. *Trans R Soc trop Med Hyg* 1926; 20: 270.

1927:

50 Leptospirosis, Tsutugamushi disease, and tropical typhus in the Federated Malay States. *Trans R Soc trop Med Hyg* 1927; 21: 283, 287.

1928:

51 Medical and sanitary services for natives in rural Africa. *Trans R Soc trop Med Hyg* 1928; 21: 461.

52 The value of roentgen rays in estimating the extent of amoebic infection of the large intestine. *Trans R Soc trop Med Hyg* 1928; 22: 214–5.

53 The surgical aspects of tropical diseases. *Trans R Soc trop Med Hyg* 1928; 22: 241.

54 The *rôle* of the spleen in the causation of haemorrhage. *Trans R Soc trop Med Hyg* 1928; 22: 326–7.

1929:

55 A case of ulcerating granuloma treated by antimony injections. *Trans R Soc trop Med Hyg* 1929; 23: 5.

56 Health problems of British Guiana. *Trans R Soc trop Med Hyg* 1929; 23: 145.

57 Blackwater fever. *Trans R Soc trop Med Hyg* 1929; 23: 382–3.

1930:

58 The etiology of yellow fever. *Trans R Soc trop Med Hyg* 1930; 23: 487.

59 The physiology of insects related to human disease. *Trans R Soc trop Med Hyg* 1930; 23: 576.

60 The morbid anatomy and histology of pellagra. *Trans R Soc trop Med Hyg* 1930; 24: 36.

61 Sprue. *Trans R Soc trop Med Hyg* 1930; 24: 184–5.

62 Pathological specimens and clinical cases. *Trans R Soc trop Med Hyg* 1930; 24:370–1.

1931:

63 *Dirofilaria immitis, Onchocerca volvulus*. Clinical cases, sprue, syphilitic myositis, beri-beri and cerebro-spinal syphilis treated with malaria. *Trans R Soc trop Med Hyg* 1931; 24: 370–1.

64 Section of a *Filaria bancrofti* in a lymphatic vessel. *Trans R Soc trop Med Hyg* 1931; 25: 3–4.

65 [*with* N H Fairley.] Gastro-jejunal-colic fistula simulating sprue: exhibition of pathological specimens. *Trans R Soc trop Med Hyg* 1931; 25: 224–5.

66 Induced malaria in England. *Trans R Soc trop Med Hyg* 1931; 24: 533–4.

67 The treatment of leprosy. *Trans R Soc trop Med Hyg* 1931; 24: 609–10.

68 Onchocerciasis in a European. *Trans R Soc trop Med Hyg* 1931; 25: 211.

69 (Review of) 'A guide to human parasitology for medical practitioners'. *Trans R Soc trop Med Hyg* 1931; 25: 215–6.

70 A case of Mediterranean leishmaniasis from Malta. *Trans R Soc trop Med Hyg* 1931; 25: 223.

1932:
71 Tryparsamide and combined treatment of Gambian sleeping sickness. *Trans R Soc trop Med Hyg* 1932; 25: 440–1.
72 The aetiology of the disease syndrome in *Wuchereria bancrofti* infections. *Trans R Soc trop Med Hyg* 1932; 26: 33–5.
73 The late Sir Ronald Ross. *Trans R Soc trop Med Hyg* 1932; 26: 203.
74 Clinical cases. *Trans R Soc trop Med Hyg* 1932; 26: 320.
75 [*with* N H Fairley.] An atypical case of amyloid disease and chronic interstitial pancreatitis. *Trans R Soc trop Med Hyg* 1932; 26: 320–2.

1933:
76 A series of tumours and microscope sections of *Onchocerca volvulus* in the tissues. *Trans R Soc trop Med Hyg* 1933; 27: 4.
77 *Entamoeba histolytica* carriers and their treatment. *Trans R Soc trop Med Hyg* 1933; 27: 127.
78 Clinical cases. *Trans R Soc trop Med Hyg* 1933; 27: 338.

1934:
79 Immunization against yellow fever. *Trans R Soc trop Med Hyg* 1934; 27: 467.
80 Clinical cases. *Trans R Soc trop Med Hyg* 1934; 28: 354.

1935:
81 Clinical cases. *Trans R Soc trop Med Hyg* 1935; 29: 358.

1936:
82 Boomerang legs and yaws in Australian aborigines. *Trans R Soc trop Med Hyg* 1936; 30: 147.

1937:
83 Clinical cases. *Trans R Soc trop Med Hyg* 1937; 30: 393.

1944:
84 Important diseases affecting West African native troops. *Trans R Soc trop Med Hyg* 1944; 37: 296.

1945:
85 Recent researches on kala-azar in India. *Trans R Soc trop Med Hyg* 1945; 39: 34.

1946:
86 Medical disorders in East Africa. *Trans R Soc trop Med Hyg* 1946; 39: 371.

1948:

87 Diseases of tropical origin in captive wild animals. *Trans R Soc trop Med Hyg* 1948; 42: 34–5.

1950:

88 Recent work on filariasis. *Trans R Soc trop Med Hyg* 1950; 44: 189–90.

Index